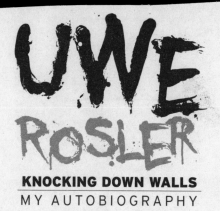

# UWE ROSLER

## KNOCKING DOWN WALLS

MY AUTOBIOGRAPHY

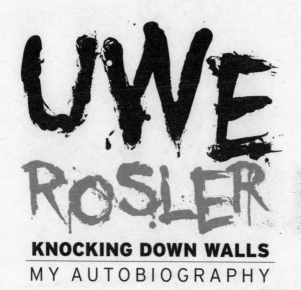

# UWE RÖSLER

## KNOCKING DOWN WALLS

MY AUTOBIOGRAPHY

Sport Media

*Dedicated to the memory my dad,*
*Horst Rosler,*
*who passed away in the summer of 2008.*

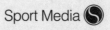

# KNOCKING DOWN WALLS

By Uwe Rosler with David Clayton

Copyright: Uwe Rosler

Published by Trinity Mirror Sport Media
Executive Editor: Ken Rogers
Publishing Director: Steve Hanrahan
Commercial Director: Will Beedles
Senior Editor: Paul Dove
Executive Art Editor: Rick Cooke
Production: Adam Oldfield, James Cleary
Design: Colin Harrison
Sales & Marketing Manager: Elizabeth Morgan
Senior Book Sales Executive: Karen Cadman
Senior Marketing Executive: Claire Brown


Paperback Edition
Published in Great Britain in 2014.
Published and produced by: Trinity Mirror Sport Media,
PO Box 48, Old Hall Street, Liverpool L69 3EB.

ISBN: 9781908695826

Photographic acknowledgements:
Uwe Rosler personal collection,
Trinity Mirror, PA Photos.


Printed and bound by CPI Group (UK) Ltd, Croydon, CR0 4YY.

# Contents

# I

# Acknowledgements

For somebody who grew up in such drab, grey surroundings, I've led a life full of colour so far and I'm very grateful for the people who have helped me achieve some of my goals in life. I'm always striving to gain knowledge and learn more, and while that is one of my strengths, it's also occasionally one of me weaknesses, too.

I know one thing. Without the help of some very special people, I wouldn't be writing a book about my life and adventures and to start, I'd like to thank my mum and my dad for all the sacrifices they made, the support they gave me no matter how far apart we were and for the love they gave me throughout my life. They taught me the values I still hold dear today and it was their understanding and desire for me to succeed that allowed me to follow my dreams.

Thank you to my mother-in-law, Grethe Hansen – I couldn't ask for a better one!

Thanks too, to Mathias Weiss who remains my best friend in Germany and was my best man at my wedding. In football, he was my mentor and advisor and he has always been there for me whenever I needed another angle on something.

My first agent, Hans Reiner Koziol, and my financial advisor Bernhard Roggenhofer, who began representing me after reunification and for looking after me at a time when I could have been left exposed and taken advantage of.

Brian Horton for taking a chance on me and Peter Beagrie for his inspiration and friendship and for someone I could never tire of being around, Gary Lee, for being a true friend and for helping me when I first came to England. Paul Walsh, the best strike partner I ever had.

Thank you to Gunnar Halle for standing by me when I needed him most and for being the brother I never had.

Thanks to Jan Aage Fjortoft for the advice he gave when I needed it the most, plus the honesty and loyalty he's shown me over the years – thank you my friend!

Otto Rehhagel for being a mentor, inspiration and a fascinating man that I can always approach for advice.

Per Matthisen for giving me the chance to move into management, for the support he gave my family when it would have been easy to turn his back. His generosity when I was fighting for my life will never be forgotten by Cecilie or me.

Thanks to Wolfgang Vöge, my agent in Germany and someone who believed in me when my stock was perhaps at an all-time low. Without him, I believe my career would have gone in a different direction.

To Joachim Streich for following his gut feeling and giving me a chance at Magdeburg and developing me into an East German international within a very short space of time – my time at the club still evokes very happy memories and I attribute that to you.

# ACKNOWLEDGEMENTS

To Paul Siguain for grounding me at Magdeburg, grounding me and taking me into his family.

I must also add a huge thank you to Dr. Grethe Lauritzen and his incredible medical staff at the hospital in Oslo, Norway. I am so grateful for the treatment and care that I received during my illness and I will forever be thankful to everyone who helped me recover.

To the City fans for all their love and support throughout my career and particularly during my illness – you lifted me when I needed it most and your continuing affection and support amazes me continually. You guys have never forgotten me and you still sing my name to this very day and I can't express how proud that makes me feel.

To David Clayton for taking the time to finalise a dream that my wife has had for so many years of me writing a book – but never seemed to find time for. David made things happen in a way that didn't affect my job in any way by being available to suit my schedule.

Thanks to the people of Brentford, to all my staff who have been so loyal and worked tirelessly and unselfishly for the past few years; thanks to Mark Warburton, who has been instrumental in my first years at Brentford and for sharing, discussing and arguing – all for the benefit of our football club and for being someone I now am proud to call a friend; a special thank you to the club's owner Matthew Benham for the support and belief and, in Matthew's case, giving me the opportunity to manage in England and for letting me run this fantastic football club.

To Bernard Halford and his family for all the fantastic support he has given me over the years. Bernard was always on hand to help me while I was a City player and when I needed anything wherever I was, he never once let me down. Bernard, when you walked up to lift the FA Cup in 2011, I had tears in my eyes – I can't think of a better tribute for someone I still think of as Mr Manchester City.

Lastly, to my beautiful wife Cecilie and my kids. Without my family I wouldn't have come anywhere near to achieving goals or being as happy as I am; my wife was my rock through my battle to survive and without her, I don't even want to think what might have become of me. I feel privileged to have spent half my life with her and I will be forever in her debt. She also gave me my two beautiful sons who are the light of my life and also raised them to be the fine young men they are today. I couldn't wish for two better boys.

# II
—

# A brief introduction...

As Uwe's wife, I consider myself lucky to be a part of his life since the summer of 1994.

His journey from a little boy in East Germany to the Bundesliga, as well as fulfilling his dream to play and work in England, has always fascinated me.

Uwe, with your drive and ambition, you have conquered the challenges of being a player and manager and I will forever admire how you used your never-say-die spirit to overcome your biggest battle, when you had to fight against cancer.

I hope you, as reader, will enjoy this book about an intelligent man who has a fascinating life story.

Thank you Uwe for being a wonderful and caring husband and dad.

LIFE WITH YOU IS NEVER BORING!

**Cecilie Rosler xxx**

# A brief introduction.

# III
—

# Prologue

My mobile phone began to ring and I started to come out of a listless sleep. For a second I didn't realise where I was. It was raining heavily outside and the wires in my arm, coupled with the pristine white sheets meant I hadn't been dreaming or, more accurately, been in the middle of a nightmare. I was still in my hospital bed recovering from the latest dose of chemotherapy and I barely had the strength to move my arms. The phone continued to ring and I picked it up and saw the name of an old friend from Manchester displayed on the screen.

"Hello...?"

There was a lot of background noise and I got the impression the caller could barely hear me.

"Uwe, can you hear it?" he shouted.

"Hear what? I can hardly hear you..."

"Listen..."

He held the phone at arm's length and I understood. My friend was calling from the City of Manchester Stadium where City were playing a home game. The City supporters were singing my name and I could hear it echoing around the ground. The news had obviously reached them and they clearly knew I was ill, but they were willing me to recover and beat the cancer that had been discovered just in time. They hadn't given up on me.

It was exactly what I needed. I ended the call and smiled for the first time in a while. I had my wife, my sons plus the support of close friends and family helping me to try and beat this. I also had 46,000 Mancunians willing me back to health.

With that kind of backing, how could I possibly fail?

# 1

# Osten ist osten

## (East is east)

Growing up in 1970s East Germany was a world away from the life the kids my age experienced in West Germany, but I wouldn't say it was any less enjoyable. Things that were maybe taken for granted in the West – nice cars, fashionable clothes, magazines and even chocolate and fruit – were rarities in the East. We lived a much simpler existence, but it was a case of what you didn't have, you didn't miss.

The Berlin Wall that divided our nation was far more than bricks and mortar – it divided cultures, families and mentalities – but it also provided me with a well-disciplined and structured path into professional football that I almost certainly wouldn't have got on the other side.

In the east, Big Brother was always watching. Our phone

calls were monitored by government agencies and the TV we watched was restricted to just two state channels, though most people could get around this by using makeshift extended aerials that meant you could watch West German TV and, best of all – and the highlight of the week – the Saturday afternoon Bundesliga highlights, where I would watch my team, Borussia Monchengladbach. Every kid who loved football would be sat in front of their TV at 6pm on a Saturday evening to see the weekend action, as well as a glimpse into another world. I was fascinated. It was like a drug: something I waited all week for and watched religiously.

The Bundesliga had so many things our own DDR-Oberliga didn't, from the glitz and glamour of some of the best players in the world to the decadence of the supporters who watched on the terraces, eating bratwurst and drinking beer.

Monchengladbach were the powerhouse of West German football in the mid-70s, winning three consecutive titles under Hans Weisweiler and later Udo Lattek with players such as Berti Vogts, Danish superstar Allan Simonsen. Even before that, in the early part of the decade, they had the brilliant Gunter Netzer in their side. That was my dream team and the one I imagined myself playing for in the schoolyard knockabouts.

My East German team was always Chemie Leipzig – the workers' team – and the lesser-known club of Leipzig, where Lokomotive had dominated for so long.

'Lok' always had the pick of the best players from the scouting and youth systems in the region. They had the best of everything and were even supported by the Communist Party on a number of levels, but I always preferred the underdogs – something that's always been in my DNA and still is to this very day.

Chemie played at the Alfred-Kunze-Sportpark – a typical English-style stadium with no running track and where the crowd were right on top of the players, all of which added extra appeal. So, if Chemie were my hometown team, Monchengladbach were my fantasy team, existing only on a TV screen, and an illegal one at that, reception courtesy of our ridiculously extended antennae. Of course, if the authorities spotted a longer-than-usual aerial on your roof, you'd be told to take it down in no uncertain terms, so it was a repressive lifestyle but, as a kid, I didn't know any different. It was just the way things were and we accepted it and got on with our lives.

I was aware that there was another world out there because I'd seen it on TV; it was like watching a movie. It wasn't reality for us and, so as long as you accepted what you saw was an alien culture and didn't question your own system, there was no real problem. Besides, everyone watched West German TV – even the Communist Party members who found watching our channels about as interesting as watching paint dry.

Privacy didn't exist and, as mentioned, even our phone calls were vetted, in that we'd have to first contact the phone company and get permission to speak with whoever it was we wanted to communicate with. Even then, the authorities would listen in.

My mum, Ingrid, had a cousin who lived in the West, but she wasn't allowed direct contact of any kind with her, so the only communication we had was when she sent a parcel for the family at Christmas. It was the highlight of Christmas Day, because we knew there would be a few gifts that were complete luxury for us – maybe milk chocolate, cake or suchlike – and it gave us a brief taste of another life. It tasted good, too. I remember one year she included a kiwi fruit in the parcel and we hadn't a clue what it was. We'd never seen one before so we didn't know if we should eat it, cook it or what. Exotic fruits were a complete mystery – we actually had to find it in an encyclopaedia before we realised what it was and that it was okay to eat it.

My home town was Starkenburg, a small village lying about 15km from the city of Altenburg, with a population of perhaps 2,000 people. My father worked in agricultural production and my mother worked in the production side of the local sausage factory, where she was the head of a laboratory.

My dad, Horst, was a very well-educated, intellectual man who was second in command of the company he worked. Neither were members of the Communist Party, which was in itself unusual for the time, but not mandatory, though my father was still involved in politics and was a member of the agricultural party, representing his local village in the district parliament of Altenburg. However, not being a Communist Party member meant there was only so far you could get in your profession – membership greased the wheels career-wise – but, if that was your choice, you accepted the consequences and got on with it.

It was through my father that my passion for football kicked in at a very early age. A very quiet and respectful person, he was, in effect, the president of the local village football club. Every weekend, he would take charge of the team and I would be alongside him, home and away.

He was a decent player himself but suffered from chronic asthma, which prevented his development at an early age, so he decided coaching was the way forward. He took just as much enjoyment from helping youngsters improve their game and running a club as he did from actually playing.

# KNOCKING DOWN WALLS

If he was laid-back and gentle, I inherited my temperament from my mother who was, in many ways, the complete opposite of my father. She worked very hard all her life and was constantly trying to develop herself and learn new working practices, particularly after the reunification of Germany, when new technology was introduced by her employers and everything completely changed. At 50, she was forced to start almost from scratch, but she didn't let anything faze her – far from it. She embraced the change and thrived in what was an exciting new world for her.

So, both my parents were an inspiration to me in their own way and I took different qualities from each. However, as time went on, they would make the ultimate sacrifice any mother or father could – effectively allowing their son to leave home at a very early age so he could follow his dreams.

I was an only child and we lived in a grey, colourless apartment block that was typical of East German housing. While it may have looked oppressive from the outside, it meant that I grew up with many friends my own age and our days would be filled with playing football, climbing trees and playing simple kids' games.

Apart from the Bundesliga, TV held little fascination for me because there was so little to watch on the two state channels. There was no internet or games consoles to keep us crouched around monitors in darkened rooms so, while it may sound alien to the youngsters of today, it was actually a very happy time for me with plenty of fresh air and exercise every day.

My parents decided they wanted a home separate from the masses and began building a house away from the apartment blocks that we eventually moved into. You were from a privileged background if you owned a detached home, but it was what they wanted and they worked hard for it, ensuring we had a better life than some.

The neighbourhood was safe – the whole country was, in reality – and after school we would play in the street or the park and do what kids are meant to do. I was into football at a very early age and was completely bitten by the bug by the age of four. My dad ensured I was part of his club and even at the age of four I'd be playing alongside kids who were a couple of years older than me – that was a pattern that would continue, to my benefit, throughout my childhood and teenage years. The minimum age was six, so it helps if you know the owner! I seldom played with my own age group and that helped me progress far quicker than my peers.

By the age of seven, maybe eight, I was selected for a local area team in Altenburg where the best of my age group had been handpicked for additional training, three times a week. As I still trained and played for my dad's village team twice a week, my ability and fitness was soon considerably more than most of the other kids and I began to stand out even more. After school – still aged only eight – I would take a 15km bus ride to the training centre where qualified coaches would take sessions.

There was a price to pay for playing and training so much and consequently; I had to leave my friends behind because my time was no longer my own. Even then, I knew what I needed to do if I wanted to succeed.

My life was school, training and sleep – but I loved it. I was laying the foundations for my future and the only caveat my parents insisted on was that my schoolwork should never take a back seat. They told me they would support me completely and take me to the games at the weekend or wherever I needed to go, but my education was equally important and if that began to suffer, things would change. It was hard because I was always so tired and after training I would still have an hour of school-work to do at home. So, whenever I did have any spare time, I just slept and tried to recover some of my energy, sometimes losing whole days at the weekend.

There were times when I was mentally and physically shat-tered because I was leaving at 7am, then jumping on a bus to go to training and returning at 8pm through the week. Was it too much? Probably, but the rewards would be worthwhile.

I did that for the next four years, so I had settled into a disci-plined routine from a very early age that would serve me well in years to come.

There was one coach in particular at my village team in Starkenburg who took great delight in bringing me back down to earth with a bang. Alois Ripel would constantly criticise parts of my game that nobody else did and it annoyed the hell out of me. Did he have a problem with me or was it that he just didn't rate me? I wasn't used to it and it got under my skin. 'You can't do this', 'that needs to improve' or 'why are you doing that when you should be doing this?' – these type of comments were continued observations of my game. It pissed me off, as I could never seem to please him.

Two or three times I told my father I was quitting and that I wanted to play for another village, but he knew the motivation behind the coach's methods and advised me to stick with it, listen to what he said and work on the areas he felt I had to im-prove on. In years to come, I came to realise that he was keeping me grounded so I could focus more and learn. It's not always the best thing to be continually told you are the best thing since sliced bread and at that stage of my development – I was a big fish in a very small pond – Alois would never allow me to rest on my laurels. He was a tough disciplinarian who I would later realise was actually crucial to my progression. In simple terms, if he didn't feel I was worth the effort, he wouldn't have bothered, so through being strict and making sure I didn't receive special treatment, he was actually pivotal in me reaching the next level.

You couldn't argue with his results, even if I wasn't always happy with his methods. For the size of our town, we were punching well above our weight and we were a really talented group of kids with a very good coach. We had made the play-offs for the highest district league in Leipzig. Nothing much ever happened in Starkenburg, so this was big news; for the home leg of the play-off there were around 2,000 people gathered around our home pitch to cheer us on. It was an experience I'll never forget. I loved playing in front of, what was for us at the time, a big crowd – it was like an actor going on stage for the first time and leaving to a huge round of applause. I was bitten and I wanted more.

I was ready for the next step. However, if I wanted to be able to take things to the next level, it would mean I'd have to make a huge sacrifice to follow my dream of becoming a footballer.

# 2

# Augen weit
# geschlossen

## (Eyes wide closed)

By the age of 11, I was playing against the best of my age group in my district, so things were progressing well, but unless I kicked on again, I would stay at the same level and perhaps never have the chance to get to where I felt I needed to be. I knew that the best players from the surrounding villages played for Attenburg, but the next level meant selecting the best of the boys from the surrounding districts – the best of the best, and the cut-off point for selection was looming. If I didn't make the intake, I'd have probably reached as far as I could go. So it was a massive relief when I discovered I'd won selection for the school of excellence in Leipzig – I was one of only 12 boys who had been chosen and it was a very select group. The only down-side was that it meant leaving home and moving to a residential building in Leipzig as the daily commute would be impossible. I would be educated, fed and looked after there – but for five days a week, I would be away from my family and would only see them at weekends. It was a huge decision for my parents because I was their only child, but they knew this was a fantastic opportunity for me. I know they agonised over the decision, and much rested on how much I wanted it to happen.

Depriving me of the chance was never discussed. They knew I would be well cared for in what would be a disciplined environment and that I would be coached after school every day at a much higher standard than I'd had so far. It was an elite group and it was what I wanted and needed. My will was so strong and I didn't consider that I'd miss home as I was already spending less and less time there. I had to do it.

People have asked me how my parents could allow me to leave the family home at such a young age and why they would even consider it, but the truth is the relationship we had made things easier. We were close, but the bond was not such that my mother and father could not survive without me and vice versa. Maybe that black and white way of thinking, thanks in no small part to my Communist upbringing, actually worked in my favour. I wanted it so badly that, despite being alone in Leipzig, they felt that was the right path for me to follow. East Germany was a safe place back then, but my mother now tells me that strong willed or not, if the same situation happened in the present day, there is no chance I would have been allowed to leave home!

So I moved out, returning only at weekends, and hit the ground running. I was a midfielder back then and was as fit as a butcher's dog (to lend an English expression), revelling in the engine room that connected defence and attack in our seven-a-side team. I was a box-to-box player and could run all day. I was confident in my own ability and maybe a touch arrogant because I'd always been the star pupil. I'd be lying if I didn't admit I had a high opinion of myself at the time. I was better and fitter than my peers, and the people of my village had made me feel I was someone special, so it was good to be among other kids my age who were just as good. From now on we would be representing Lokomotive Leipzig whenever we played, as the school was a feeder for their junior teams. It was drummed into us from a very early age that we represented the club and in many ways we were being groomed to be politicians in tracksuits.

I soon settled in and was given a room with two other boys my age – Mathias Paske, who came from Schwerin in the north, and Ingo Saager. They became my family and the brothers I'd never had. We got along well, played football together, ate together and lived in each other's pockets for the next four years.

I was learning to stand on my own two feet, but it was a disciplined lifestyle. We had to make sure our room was perfect or risk getting a mark against us. It was not unlike a military school in that respect, and if the bathroom was dirty, the toilets left unclean or the beds unmade, you were chastised and like everything else we did, it encouraged a competitive edge. The school of excellence catered for all sports and there were just as many track and field athletes, swimmers, weightlifters, marksmen, volleyball and handball players and gymnasts as there were footballers. It was the best of the best from the region that had Leipzig as its capital, but there was a harsher side to life there.

It had a fascinating food system, too. You were given coloured tokens for meal times – red, green and blue. Red was only for world and Olympic champions – they had the best food of everyone on the campus and instead of one steak, they would get two, plus a better selection of vegetables and fruit. Depending on where you were in the pyramid, you were allotted a token that matched where you were development-wise, so we had blue tokens – the basic food programme, which was still good, but a long way short of what a red token would get you. We knew that if we worked hard, one day we could be on the red tokens, too, so from the moment we arrived, we were reminded that we had targets to reach if we wanted to be the best.

You could beat the system on occasions. For the evening meals between 5pm and 8pm, my pals and I would arrive early at the food hall because our training was only a couple of hours in the afternoon. People would arrive at all sorts of times, depending on their training regimes. We knew that if we ate fast enough, we could go to the back of the queue and eat the same meal again. Wolfing down food would become a habit I still have to this day, but it was worth it!

If your education was not up to standard, you wouldn't be accepted – except in very rare cases where the talent was so exceptional they turned a blind eye to the normal rules of enrolment. This was private education of the highest standard that included board, schooling and the best food you could get, so they could afford to be choosy. My parents didn't have to pay a single penny – it all came from the local government, so the selection process was strict and at times unforgiving.

The thinking was that by finding the most talented and promising kids across East Germany, and then ensuring they were nurtured accordingly, it would result in the country producing champions in sport – the only platform we could compete on a level footing in and win medals in major competitions such as the Olympics, world championships or whatever. We were being groomed and channelled into a system that bred champions and as a result, it was roundly criticised for many years by other nations. However, the truth is that the East German government was maybe 30 years ahead of everyone else because where do you find the most talented kids and future sports stars of today? In similar nurturing systems, schools of excellence and academies around the world.

Yet there was a darker side to this privileged life, with certain youngsters developing at unnatural rates because of the steroids they were being given. Female swimmers would change dramatically over the course of a few years, becoming more powerful and having speaking voices that were as deep as the men. The systematic doping to enhance certain groups was part of our culture, but as a kid, you don't think like that and I never questioned the treatment of others because it all seemed part of the process. One thing I can categorically say was that the doping didn't extend to football, or at least, I never saw any evidence to suggest as much.

Each year your progress would be reviewed and if you didn't make the cut, you would be released back to normal everyday life and this was the case for the first four years because 16 was the cut-off age when a final decision was taken. I was 15 and was a late developer, so while other boys were getting stronger and taller and becoming young men, I wasn't and things were reaching a critical point.

I was, by that time, being coached as a striker and scored

plenty of goals for the team initially, but my lack of physical development was holding me back and it was getting harder and harder for me to make an impression in games. I lost the captaincy and people started to wonder why I was starting to stand still – had I already peaked, as many kids do at that age and begun to flat-line? It couldn't have happened at a worse time because my coach, Roland Freyer, had pretty much made his mind up that I wasn't up to it and wanted me out – but I was lucky.

Thomas Matheja, the Leipzig Under-17s coach, along with a coach we knew as Dr. Kirsche, who ran the Under-18s, both saw something in me that they felt they could nurture and it was my good fortune that they were ultimately responsible for bringing young players through to the senior squad. There were only five players going to the next level and the remainder would be released – the five had been chosen, but Matheja and Dr. Kirsche decided to ignore Freyer's recommendation and they made an extra place for me. They took a gamble and without their belief and insistence, I'd have joined the scrapheap before my 16th birthday. Thankfully, it didn't come to that. Ingo and Mathias had made it through as well so I still had my two adopted brothers alongside me, though I knew that would end at some point – we all did. The whole process was about survival of the fittest and I have always believed I am a born survivor – a quality that would effectively save my life in later years.

I now felt that I was at last on my way. All the long journeys, the time away from my family and hard work had all paid off. Now I had to repay the faith my new coach had shown in me, and quickly. There was still a mountain to climb and the clock was ticking…

# 3

# Befasst sich mit dem Teufel

## (Deals with the Devil)

It was a relief when my shirt became tighter, my trousers became too short and I went up a couple of boot sizes within a few months as I hit a rapid growth spurt around my 16th birthday. Before long I had won my place back in the team and continued to progress as a player. In many ways, footballers have two careers – the one during the schoolboy years and then the youth and adult period and, for some, it's a bit of lottery. I was lucky that I had experienced coaches who had seen it all before, but there will be countless others who didn't make it because their coach maybe didn't understand that everyone developed at their own rate and lost patience. Though I didn't feel I had a second chance, I knew what it felt to have been on the border-line and I didn't want to repeat that uncertainty again.

I was scoring goals again and grew 12 centimetres in height inside a year. As a result, I had one or two injuries that season which were literally down to growing pains, but by the age of 18, everything seemed to have evened out and I had done well enough to win selection for the East Germany national Under-18s, and I couldn't have felt more proud.

I'd made good friends with a number of older players at Lo-komotive who no longer lived at the halls of residence and instead had a private apartment, which was obviously much more appealing. I unofficially moved in with them, all of which opened up a completely new world that involved girls, nightlife and drink, though I was focused enough not to go crazy.

I had my eyes opened and I loved being in the company of the older lads who ranged between 18 and 21. I have always tried to stretch myself in that respect. I was like a sponge, absorbing everything and broadening my horizons while making my way through the Lokomotive youth ranks.

Football was always my driving force, but I discovered disco-theques and girls and life was good. In fairness, I'd had my first drink as a 15-year-old at the halls of residence where we'd been allowed to stay out till 10pm one night of the week, so I wasn't completely green. Life on the edge!

Alcohol was very cheap and there was a strategy from the gov-ernment so people would drink more and complain less! There was a drinking culture, but not one that was out of control – more for recreational purposes than anything else. Forget cars, holi-days, houses, fruit or expensive clothes – we were allowed to have the basics to live – meat, vegetables, potatoes and cheap booze.

That was all another world as far as I was concerned as I got closer to the senior squad. Ingo was still by my side but Mathias Paske had been released and I would never see him again, which was a shame, but I had to move on with my life.

East German football had its critics, but the system for youth football was second to none and the integration from top level to youth was superb. On a matchday, if the senior team was at home to Dynamo Dresden, the Under-16s would kick off on pitches next to the stadium at 11am, and then straight after the Under-18s would occasionally play in the main stadium before the senior side kicked off. A lot depended on the state of the pitch and the weather being good, but if everything was fine, you could be playing in front of crowds of 20,000, which was an amazing experience for a kid and the incentive it gave you to succeed was incalculable, giving you a taste of one possible future. The first-team would go and warm up on a pitch near the stadium while the younger lads played their game as the crowd filtered in.

Pulling on that East German Under-18s national team shirt was a very proud experience for me and it felt like a reward for 10 years of hard work. The politicians in tracksuits theory was never truer than when you represented your country because we were junior diplomats flying the flag for our nation and, from the government's perspective, for communism, too. Playing for your country at any level is a massive thing for any footballer – or at least it should be – and it meant everything to me. It also meant I was on track and heading in the right direction, so long as I kept doing what I did.

I signed my first contract with Leipzig, aged 18, in 1987. I didn't get paid because you were offered the chance of an apprenticeship as either a mechanic or an electrician because Lokomotive's background is in the railways of the east, and if all else failed, you could have a career working in the rail industry instead. There was an option to study medicine – which I wasn't smart enough to do – or continue for another three years with your education, which is the path I chose because I had no interest in either of the apprenticeships on offer. Trust me, if I didn't make it, the last thing I wanted to do was repair train engines. I elected to study sports and physical education because I always intended becoming a coach at some point. I received 150 East German marks per month through the apprenticeship – about 10 euros – not a fortune by any stretch of the imagination and a little different from the talented teenagers of today, but I was happy enough.

But there were lows as well as highs. Mixing with the first-team was something I maybe wasn't quite ready to do and I handled things badly after a humiliating episode that left me feeling totally crushed. I was no longer one of the elite few who had overcome numerous hurdles to get to this point; now I was just a youth player promoted to the senior squad – a grunt with everything to prove, and the older pros had seen us come and go by the bucket-load. Lok were a very strong team and had reached the final of the European Cup Winners' Cup the previous May, losing 1-0 to Ajax in Athens. I would be trying to force my way into one of the best teams in Europe at that time and it was both daunting and exciting for a kid my age.

I'd come a long way and was proud of my journey from my village team all the way through to Lokomotive Leipzig's senior squad, but everything turned sour pretty quickly. At the first day of pre-season training for the 1987/88 campaign, the whole squad were together for the first time, including maybe eight East German internationals and another four Under-21 internationals. It was a little intimidating to say the least.

The assistant coach, Gunter Böhme, gathered everyone together and he said that I, plus two other guys around the same age, were joining the squad. Then he looked at me and said: "By the way, this is Uwe Rosler, but don't worry, he will never make it…" He had a reputation for trying to break new players and if they came through it, they would have a real chance, but I was devastated and reduced to tears in front of so many players I looked up to, all of whom were laughing. It was like one of those nightmares you wake up from sweating, relieved to discover it was just a bad dream – only it wasn't.

I'd gone there with such nervous energy and enthusiasm, wanting to show what I was capable of, and instead I felt humiliated and I wanted some payback – I'd always had a temper on me but I had to wait for the right moment to even the scores. Two days later, I got the chance. We were playing a popular small-sided game with 5 v 2 in a coned-off box and Gunter Böhme was in the team against me. As the ball went towards him, I lunged in and caught him high on his knee, leaving a 30cm open wound. I didn't say anything, but that tackle alone said "Don't fuck with me." In my eyes it was justified, but it was a naïve thing to do and there was no way back, with our relationship already irreversibly damaged.

I gained some respect from the older players, but my card had already been marked and that incident would stay in the mind of both the coach and the manager. I got my head down after that and stayed out of trouble as best I could

The season finally began in July and I did well enough in pre-season to be named as substitute for the fourth game of the season against Hansa Rostock – it was 29th August, 1987, and I came on during the second half, so I was off and running at senior level.

My second game was even more memorable and again I came on as a second-half sub against Olympique Marseille in the second round, first leg of the UEFA Cup. There were around 80,000 people in Leipzig's main stadium where the national team also played. Lok had a smaller ground they used for league games, but this was incredible and I had to pinch myself that this was all happening so quickly. I suppose if I'd needed reminding how big this club was, that game, the crowd and the expectation that was almost tangible, brought everything home to me. I was a wet-behind-the-ears youngster who was suddenly up against some of the biggest starts in European football, many of whom had been at the 1986 World Cup just a year before. Stellar names such as Joseph Bell, Jean-Pierre Papin, Jean-François Domergue, Bernard Genghini, German legends Karlheinz Forster and Klaus Allofs, so it was a terrific experience and gave me a glimpse of the career I could have if I continued to believe in myself and work hard.

I was up against the man-mountain that was Yvon Le Roux, but I held my own even if I didn't manage to get on the scoresheet. It ended 0-0 and it was a proud night for the Rosler family, with my mum and dad in the crowd that night. Not long after that high, I found myself in an agonising situation that, perhaps more than anything else, demonstrates how different life was in East Germany before reunification.

It was unnerving, unsettling and morally corrupt, but all-too common in the days before reunification. I was still doing my studies as part of the three years extra studying programme in sport that I had to undertake. On one unremarkable afternoon, I received a visit from a Lokomotive polite (pronounced 'poleet') officer – a representative of the communist party who was their eyes and ears at each football club. He came to my school to see me, which was very unusual in itself. He asked me if we could talk somewhere quiet and so we went to the director's office, where he asked me what I was doing next. I told him I had one more lesson and then was off to training.

"No, no," he said. "You don't have to come to training today. Somebody will pick you up from the front of the school at 4pm. Don't be late."

I asked who it was I was to meet and he told me I didn't need to know who or why, just to be there when the car arrived. I immediately feared that I was about to meet the East German secret police – the Stasi – not dissimilar to the Russian KGB and it could only mean something bad was about to happen. In the Easter Bloc you never knew when you might receive a visit from them, all you knew was it was better when they were speaking to someone other than you. They were a secret department of the government with a reputation for making offers that could not be refused. They were always watching people who they thought might be speaking out of turn or planning to flee the country. People were always looking over their shoulder and loose tongues could ruin careers of individuals and their family members if they happened to find out.

So why did they want to talk to me? I wondered if my dad had drunk too much in the pub one night and spoke his mind about the government. The Stasi had informants everywhere and you didn't really know who you could trust and who you couldn't, all of which bred suspicion and a sense of paranoia. I was someone the government had already invested a lot of time and money on and I was also something of a risk because I travelled abroad occasionally with the East Germany Under-21 team. Four or five players had already defected to the west, so we were always under scrutiny.

I was terrified and they knew I would be terrified. They had the power to make sure I never played football again while ending the jobs of my mother and father, too. If they wanted, they had the power to send me to serve 18 months in the army and not be allowed to train, so I would effectively be finished or, at best, struggling to rebuild my career. My future was totally in their hands.

Two guys picked me up in a Wartbug 311 and drove me through Leipzig and then stopped, got out of that car and into another, presumably in case we were being followed. We then continued the journey and travelled a long way – at least it seemed a long way – before we arrived at the world-renowned Deutsche Hochschule für Körperkultur University in Leipzig – a famous East German academy that had a reputation for excellence that was renowned worldwide.

I got out and went into the building where I was led to a big office where there was one desk, a high ceiling, one small window and two Stasi officers waiting. It was a typical good cop, bad cop routine with one guy walking around asking if I was okay or if I wanted a coffee, while the other guy just sat there looking stern, speaking only occasionally. My nerves had completely gone and I just wanted it to be over, whatever 'it' was. Finally, the stern guy said: "So you've been to Sweden with Lokomotive Leipzig? And to France as well?"

I said I had.

He nodded. "Good, good. And while you were away, there were some East Germans who talked to the players at the hotel bar. Do you remember that?"

I did remember that. There was a group of Lokomotive fans who now lived abroad and followed the club around Europe and after a time, they became familiar to the players who talked with them after matches. These were people who had moved on from East Germany by one mean or another. You left East Germany only one of a few ways – you could run or take the official way out, which could have been because of relatives living elsewhere, financial incentives for the government or very low level individuals who were so far off the radar they weren't considered to be the slightest threat. Because they were living a new life in the west, the government considered them to be a threat – would they try and entice the players to maybe make a similar move? When they chatted at the bar, what had been said? These were things the Stasi needed to know and because clearly none of their informers had provided the necessary information, they were trying 'alternative' methods.

I could see where this was heading. "You know what?" I said, "I'm a young player and after I'd eaten I went straight to bed. I didn't see or hear anything."

The trip to Marseille had been interesting but there wasn't even a hint of anything unusual, but when we had travelled to Sweden, I'd done something that had clearly put the wind up our ever-watchful polite officer. East Germany was grey – grey buildings, grey cars and people even wore grey clothing. There was a distinct lack of colour in our lives so Sweden was a breath of fresh air. From the moment we got off the plane, I was fascinated with the country. Beautiful green hills and fauna, blue skies, fresh clean air and houses brightly coloured in red, green white and blue. It was the least grey place I'd ever been to and it couldn't have been more different from the dreary streets and cities back home. I instantly fell in love with Scandinavia and that would come back to me in later years. Our guide invited us all back to his house for drinks and a barbecue and in his garage he had a Harley Davidson. I was the only player in the Lok team who had a motorbike at that time – everyone else had a car – so I had a particular interest in the Harley and the guy could probably see my eyes bulging out of their sockets.

"Ah, my friend," he said. "Would you like a ride on it?"

Now bear in mind I was one of the younger players and supposed to keep quiet and maintain a low profile, but this was an offer I couldn't refuse.

"Could I?" I said. He tossed me the keys and told me to start it up. I sat on that comfortable seat and turned the engine over – it purred just like I knew it would, and then I set off for a ride around the block. The other players looked stunned and the polite officer looked terrified, as did our club officials who had vouched that the trip was absolutely watertight. The problem was, I got lost and couldn't find my way back! They must have thought I had headed for the hills and wasn't coming back, but although the feeling of freedom in such beautiful surrounds was very liberating, I never considered anything but a quick trip around the block. Eventually, I found my way back and even though I was only gone for 20 minutes or so, I received such a bollocking on my return that my pleasant memory soon faded into nothing. No wonder the Stasi were asking me questions.

"Ah, okay," he said. "So things are going well for you? You are enjoying playing for Lokomotive?"

I said that I loved it and everything was going really well, mentioning playing in the game against Marseille as I tried to stay chatty and friendly.

"And do you want to continue playing for them?" the stern one said.

"Of course," I replied.

"Then you must work with us."

There it was. The charade was over and it was exactly as I'd dreaded. The whole point of the exercise was that they wanted me to become an informant, letting them know what the players were talking about or if any of them had any plans to take any 'long holidays' – the kind that you didn't need a return ticket for.

I didn't say anything, and just kept quiet.

"You are very good at school," he continued, "and have interesting views during political discussions. You are an ambitious player with a great future, but you have to work with us, Rosler."

I shifted nervously. "I just want to play football and do my schooling, that's all. I don't want any trouble."

The stern guy shook his head. "It's not working. You are either with us or against us, and if you are against us, you are finished. You will not play for the national team, you won't play for Lokomotive again and your career will be over. We have your destiny in this hand," he added, clinching his fist. "So what is your decision? Be somebody or nobody?"

Football was my life and it was all I wanted to do – I couldn't imagine living without it. I tried to be clever and buy myself some time. "Can I think about it? This is a massive decision for me. I need to speak with my parents about this…"

"No!" he shouted, pushing a piece of paper in front of me. "You can't talk to anyone about our meeting – not your parents or your friends, nobody. Do you understand? Now you must to sign this."

I glanced down at it. It said words to the effect that I had never met these people, and that this meeting had never happened, so I did as I was asked. I was then allowed to leave and headed straight back to Starkenburg to visit my parents. It was a Friday evening so they knew straight away that something wasn't right. I wondered why they'd made me sign that document – was it so they had a record of my signature? I was uncomfortable about the whole situation.

My father asked what was wrong, what had I done? I told him I couldn't tell him and that I had been sworn to secrecy, but of course eventually I did. "The Stasi want me to keep them informed about the first-team players and what they are saying and doing. Who they talk to when we go abroad, how much do they drink and if they are thinking of using one of the trips away to stay in that country. I don't want to do it; I just want to play football."

I knew my dad would know what to do and he gave me the best advice possible. "The only chance for you to get out of this Uwe is to speak to the manager of Lokomotive. He will know what the best solution is."

I had signed the paper and I knew the Stasi came to home games, yet I'd already told my father and now I was to tell my manager, too. It was a gamble that could easily backfire and I didn't sleep a wink that night as I thought through all the possible consequences of my actions. The following day I went to training and I was terrible, so much so that the manager came across and asked me what was wrong. I told him I had a problem that I couldn't tell him about and that I probably wouldn't be able to play football for him or anyone anymore.

"You can tell me anything," he said.

I couldn't carry the burden around any longer so I told him that I'd been asked to do something I didn't want to do and I think he knew straight away what I was talking about and who was behind it.

"Those fucking arseholes!" he shouted. "They have no right to bother my players!"

He was in a rage but eventually he composed himself, took a deep sigh and told me he would sort this out. He called the club's CEO and said he must warn the Stasi away and that they had to leave his players alone. "They are arseholes and my players are not politicians! End this now!" He slammed the phone down and told me to forget about it.

I looked at him in total disbelief. "And now I'm fucked," I said. "My dad knows, you know and now the CEO knows so soon the Stasi will know I have spoken about this."

"No, no," he said, "coming to me was the best thing you could have done. Don't worry about this anymore, Uwe, just do your studies and play football."

The next few weeks were unbearable and I waited for a visit or a phone call, but it didn't come. Eventually, I thought that it might have been sorted somehow, but I wasn't completely certain. I carried on as normal because that was all I could do, but if I hadn't sought advice, I really don't know what would have happened because I could never have done their dirty work. I was a footballer, not a spy nor an informant.

Returning to some kind of normality, I was surprised when

I was named as sub for the opening league games, coming off the bench in the first four matches, so things were going well and I thought that was that. After a league game for Lok on the Saturday, I played for the second-team, who were playing my hometown team of Attenburg away, which was a special game for me. There were maybe 6,000 people there, such was the pull of Lokomotive Leipzig, but things went badly and I was targeted throughout the game by one guy who was kicking me, pulling my shirt and generally trying to wind me up from the start. Eventually I went up for a header and elbowed him in the face as I jumped. I'd had enough, but the referee saw the incident and showed me a straight red card. Any progress I'd made counted for nothing because in my first six weeks, I'd injured the assistant coach and now I'd let a defender get inside my head. How could they trust a temperamental 18-year-old not to do it again? Next time maybe something I did would cost us the game? I was banned for eight weeks and though I trained with the seniors, the club were already making plans to move me on. I couldn't turn back the clock and I was raw and inexperienced, but I still wonder if things might have turned out differently had I not suffered such humiliation on my first day. I'd worked hard and been part of Lokomotive's academy for six years, leaving my family and friends behind, but it had taken me just six weeks to undo everything I'd worked so hard for.

As a footnote, during my ban I would watch the home games from the players' VIP area and on one occasion, the two Stasi agents that had dealt with me turned up. They didn't say a thing and just stared at me before I left the room, suitably disturbed by their presence. Maybe I had won after all, but they certainly let me know they were still around, but clearly they'd been told to back off. My manager had been right – arseholes.

Despite my resistance, in later years I would discover that fou or five players I knew and respected had been working for the Stasi all along. Their information funded a different lifestyle that bought them new homes, cars and wealth, but when Germany reunified, the papers were released and they were named and shamed, though I knew that some of them would have done what they did through sheer panic. I must admit, even though I knew I'd signed a fairly harmless piece of paper when they'd interrogated me, the way they worked, there was a nagging doubt that underneath that paper there was another claiming I was a Stasi informant. Thankfully that wasn't the case and I was just glad the whole sorry episode was finally behind me and that I could get on with my career, though it didn't seem as though it would be with Lokomotive Leipzig.

Indirectly, my indiscretions on the pitch led to a move I was more than happy to agree to, as Lok informed me I was being loaned out to Chemie Leipzig, the team I'd supported as a boy. Though I didn't know it at the time, I would never play for Lokomotive again.

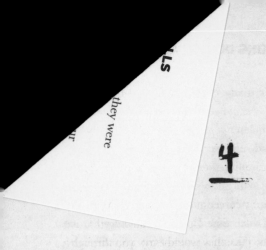
they were

# 4

# Lichter der
# Stadt

## (City Lights)

Moving to Chemie was exactly as I'd hoped. I felt a lot of empathy with the club who had always been the poor relations of Leipzig. The two sets of fans hated each other and there was the added spice that a number of the Chemie squad – including myself – had been released or moved on by Lokomotive and so felt they had something to prove. It made for a good camaraderie among the lads who enjoyed – shall we say – a vibrant social scene as well.

Things went okay if not fantastically well, but the important thing was I was playing every week and learning to play men's football, which was crucial for my development. I'd also kept my place in the East Germany Under-21 team where I felt I performed really well. I finally felt things were moving in the right direction for my career.

Playing for my boyhood club added something extra to my game and I think it came through in my football, too. I soon formed a strong bond with the players and the fans, something I'd try and do throughout my career at each club I represented. I tried to give everything each time I played, knowing that if you had the backing of the fans, they would carry you through any difficult periods you might encounter. The DDR-Liga – the second tier of East German football – meant we were regularly up against some tough, experienced opponents, and as a kid with a reputation for losing my head, I was targeted for 'special attention' on more than one occasion, with word getting around that I'd been ushered out of Lok for reasons not necessarily due to lack of ability. I needed that gritty, tough grounding, and playing in an environment where it was the survival of the fittest helped me grow up quickly.

I'd spent just one season with Chemie, scoring six goals in 27 appearances, and was surprised when Lok recalled me because I thought my time there was over. It turned out I was right, too. This wasn't a recall to challenge for their first-team. Nothing had really changed; it was just that my stock had risen. I'd proved I could hold my own and I now had value in the transfer market, so they could get me off their books once and for all, as well as getting a financial return of some sort.

Matthias Weiss became my mentor at Chemie and he was a fantastic influence for me, somebody I became very close to. I was so happy there that I think he knew I would probably stay at the club to my own detriment. Joachim Streich, the manager of FC Magdeburg, had come to watch me after one particular game and I was told he wanted to meet me. In the shower, I asked Matthias what I should do because Magdeburg seemed keen to take me.

He was the captain of the team and we had a good chance of winning promotion, but he still said: "Uwe, when you want to achieve something in life, you have to go."

He could have been selfish and advised me to stay, but he didn't, and it was the start of a lifelong friendship that remains strong to this day.

I'd only been back at Lok for a few weeks when Magdeburg came back for me. It was initially a loan deal and I moved there in January 1989. They were fighting relegation in the Oberliga and had a good, young team that I felt could really be of benefit to me. The deal worked well for all parties as I played my part in helping them beat the drop. Lok wanted a Magdeburg player – Damian Halata – a Polish-born striker who was also an East German international and something of a Magdeburg legend. He'd been at the club for eight years and decided it was the right time to move on, so an exchange deal was agreed between Lok and Magdeburg, finally allowing me to sever my ties with Leipzig for good. It was decent business all round – both clubs were happy with the deal – but I wasn't quite finished with my old nemesis Gunter Böhme, the assistant coach at Lok who had humiliated me on my first day with the senior squad.

As often seems to happen in football, one of my first games as a Magdeburg player was away to Lokomotive and, late on in the game, the ball fell to me in the box and I tucked it away for what proved to be the winning goal. Unable to control my emotions, and if I'm honest, not particularly wanting to, I ran halfway up the pitch to the Lok bench and flipped Gunter the middle finger. It felt good at the time and, in truth, I don't regret what I did. But, of course, it was foolish because it wasn't exactly going to go unnoticed and caused a scandal in East German football. The game was live on TV so the whole country knew about what had happened. There had never been anything like that seen before on TV, and after the game a polite officer came into our dressing room and demanded I make an immediate apology. I suppose my actions confirmed everything Lok had suspected about my temperament, but all my anger was aimed at Gunter – I don't think I could have made that any more obvious.

The East German newspapers didn't mention a thing because everything was always neutral and professional, with no speculation or gossip – just straight reporting and nothing else. They gave a match report, marked you out of 10 and that was it – in fact, I was even in the team of the week, so had the cameras not been there, it would have been like nothing had ever happened. Reluctantly, I apologised through the media and I explained my actions were not aimed at Lokomotive, who had helped me get to where I wanted to be and that I liked the club, the manager and the players – it was all aimed at Gunter. It didn't do me any favours, but that's who I was and I couldn't change my nature, nor did I want to.

Many years later, I took part in a charity game and Gunter was in charge of the opposition. After the match he came to see me and he told me that what I'd done all those years ago had really troubled him since. "Why did you do that Uwe? I've never understood."

"I did it because of how you treated me on my first day at Lok," I told him.

"But I did that to all the young players, Uwe."

"But you could have destroyed me…"

"Yes, but look where you are today."

"Maybe Gunter, but how many more didn't get as far as I did because they were too crushed by your comments?"

We parted on friendly terms and I was happy to have laid that particular moment to rest.

Life at Magdeburg was great, and I really came into my own at the Ernst-Grube-Stadion. I was scoring goals, playing really well and I felt at home. For me, they were the right club at the right time and things started to click because I had the right players around me and I was maybe the missing link in their team. In Dirk Heyne, Dirk Stahmann and Wolfgang 'Maxe' Steinbach, I had three seasoned pros to look up to and learn off. Wolfgang was my mentor in many ways. He was 35 and nearing the end of his career, but he was still a magnificent footballer – a genius, in fact. He was like an American football quarterback pulling the strings. He didn't move much but he could pick a pass out and put the ball on a sixpence.

We had a fantastic team with the right mix of youth and experience, with players coming through such as Markus Wuckel – my strike partner – Stefan Minkwitz, Dirk Schuster and my good friend, Jens Landrath. We had a lot of energy, talent and hunger and that's why we complemented each other so well.

Wolfgang pulled the strings in midfield and together with the two Dirks, they made me look good and the goals started to come. I needed those players to help me move to the next level. Wolfgang was instrumental in my progression because he made so many goals for me, and technically he was one of the best players I ever played with. But he also had an edge to his game, which I liked. We were training on one occasion and I went in for a tackle with him and won the ball. Wolfgang shouted to stop the session.

"Never do that again."

"Why? I asked. "I got the ball."

"I could have broken your leg. In a 50-50 situation like that, you should go over the ball, connect with his shin and collect the ball."

That stuck in my mind for the rest of my career, and I'm certain I would have broken my leg had I continued to go in for challenges as I had. I was also fortunate to have an East Germany legend as my manager. Joachim Streich has scored 229 goals in 378 appearances during a magnificent playing career and his international record – 55 goals in 102 appearances – spoke for itself.

Outside of our country, he was relatively unknown, but in East Germany he was a superstar. I learned more from the advice and informal chats we had in his office than I did from anyone else throughout my career. He made me feel 10 feet tall, believed in me and offered me simple suggestions to help me improve. He knew how to get the best out of me and when he took shooting drills with the keepers it was clear that he'd lost nothing other than perhaps the speed he had at his peak.

I had more confidence than I'd ever had before and I remember nipping into his office in between training sessions to speak to him on more than one occasion. He was so relaxed, he sometimes even enjoyed a beer and a cigarette over our chats – not that he ever offered me a drink (of course I probably would have refused it…). He talked to me about every aspect of the game and before long, I would have run through brick walls for him. It seemed the sky was the limit and all Joachim had done was talk me up, tell me that he thought I was a great player and showed me areas where I could become even better. He told me he had a gut instinct about me, which is why he'd taken me to Magdeburg and he always went with his instincts.

As a group, we worked hard and we played hard. We enjoyed our time on and off the pitch and there were plenty of nights out along the way. The majority of us were young and single and we made the most of our bachelorhood, with Saturday the big night out. It was the one night of the week when we all released the pressure that had built up during the week. Sundays would be a rest day and then the build up to the next match would begin all over again. I'd always ease into the week and step up gradually to Friday, when I'd be like a coiled spring. Everyone had their own methods of preparation but that's what worked for me.

I'd put all thoughts of the Stasi behind me and had moved on with my career, but there was a curious trip at the start of the 1989/90 season that made me think back to that time. We were drawn against Bayer Uerdingen from West Germany in the Intertoto Cup, and they had a 20-year-old Danish talent called Brian Laudrup making his debut for them that day. Just before we left for the journey across the border, the CEO of Magdeburg received a phone call from the Stasi who told him: "Rosler can't go."

For me, playing a Bundesliga side was the highlight of the year because we were up against teams we only ever saw on TV – plus, as a bonus we were paid 25 West German marks each day, which was a fortune for us. It was a trip everyone wanted to go on, so to be told I couldn't, and also not be given a reason, was cruel in the extreme. Maybe the Stasi were having the last laugh after all?

The CEO told them I was one of the club's best players and I was needed for that game, which was important not only to Magdeburg, but for all of East Germany. They were unrepentant. "No," they said. "His best friend has disappeared. Leave him behind."

It transpired that I did have a friend who was playing for a club near my home town and, like us, they were also in the Intertoto Cup. It seemed he'd taken his chance for a new life when his team went abroad and now they assumed I would do the same thing, because I would also have an opportunity to break free of the shackles and red tape that made our lives so claustrophobic at times.

The Stasi were convinced my friend and I had an agreement of some kind and as he'd already fled, they wanted to keep me back as a precaution. Of course, I hadn't spoken to him for some time and knew nothing of his plans, but the authorities weren't interested in what I had to say. My CEO, however, did have some clout and he refused to give up. He fought for me and somehow got me on the trip – I'm not sure what personal guarantees he made on my behalf, but I was grateful and relieved. After the game, we were heading for Krefeld on the coach, enjoying a few beers along the way back after a 1-1 draw. We were approaching a motorway service station in West Germany to refuel and curiously, as we pulled in, my mentor, Wolfgang Steinbach, leaned over to me and said: "How about when we stop, we go to the toilet and just disappear?!"

He was my idol and though it was only said for a laugh, the way we'd been conditioned meant you were never 100 per cent sure about anything. Maybe he was trying to give me a push to flee to the west, but I'm not sure either way. If I'd have said I did want to go, I think he probably would have told me to go while I had the chance. Of course, we stayed on the coach and returned home, but the opportunity was there. It would have been nice to get one over on the Stasi, but it wasn't what I really wanted at that point and if the CEO had vouched for me, I would have dropped him right in it. Besides, my parents would have been made to suffer and after all the sacrifices they had already made for me, I wasn't about to let them down. Maybe Wolfgang was ready but didn't want to go alone? I don't think I'll ever really know.

# 5

# Ein weiterer Stein in der Mauer?

## (Another brick in The Wall?)

Spying, informers, defectors, suspicion and paranoia – just a way of life for every East German, but there was growing civil unrest in my country and it was peaking at exactly the wrong time for my career, which sounds a little selfish, I know. I'd started to play for my country in 1989 and won my first full cap against Kuwait. We were also in with a great chance of making the 1990 World Cup in Italy, and were second in our qualifying group with one match remaining. Our final game was in Vienna against Austria and if we drew, we'd guarantee automatic qualification, which was a massive thing for our country. Our coach was Eduard Geyer, also the boss of Dynamo Dresden and we were determined to give ourselves the best possible chance to get through.

It was such an important game that the Oberliga was suspended for two weeks to give the national team plenty of time to prepare properly, and so we were based in Leipzig and trained at the national stadium behind closed doors. During this period, we found ourselves in the middle of a potentially horrific situation as we prepared for our trip to Austria.

The protests in Leipzig had begun a few weeks earlier at the Nikolai Church, where Parson Christian Fuhrer had been publicly advocating free speech, freedom of thinking and liberty. 'The Monday Demonstrations', as they became known, were attracting larger crowds each time. One hundred the first week, one thousand the next, 10 thousand the week after and eventually they relocated to Karl Mark Square, where close to 100,000 gathered in a peaceful protest chanting 'We are the People! We are the People!' It was an unprecedented public show of defiance as our people finally found their voice.

We were in the middle of a revolution and with all the civil unrest, our concentration couldn't help but be affected. As the day of the game approached, the biggest protest yet hit the streets of Leipzig. It was a tinderbox, ready to explode at any moment because it seemed only a matter of time before the security forces took action. Then, as we relaxed at our team hotel, a police chief came in and gave a big speech about how this was an amazing chance for East Germany and how important the game was to everybody. Chillingly, he then added: "And don't worry about the protests because tonight it will end. We have surrounded Leipzig centre and will move in with the military and end it once and for all!"

He said it as though he was expecting us to stand up and cheer him at the end. I couldn't believe what I was hearing. He added to warn our families and friends to stay away from Leipzig because of what was going to happen so, understandably, our minds were anywhere but on the approaching football match. Later, we discovered that the leader of the Communist Party in Leipzig held the military back and didn't follow the orders he'd been given, saving the lives of thousands of innocent people. Thank God. A week passed before 320,000 people gathered in Karl Marx Square, and three weeks later the Berlin Wall was finally torn down. It was the end of life as we knew it as our country headed towards a bright, free future.

What amazed me was that before that happened, football agents from West Germany suddenly appeared and based themselves close to our training camp. It was clear the communist era was coming to an end so they wanted to move quickly to secure the best players for West German clubs. Our official status was that we were amateurs – even though we were actually very well paid – but we were entering a totally new world where some very talented footballers would be available for nothing. We were getting phone calls in our rooms offering big contracts and a new life in the West.

Football had become a side issue but we still had a massive game to play. Two players were cut from the senior side and I was one of them, so would instead appear for the Under-21s. We all travelled together to Austria where, given the disruption back home, it was no surprise the team lost 3-0. We won our game the night before 1-0 to finish second in our group, but the senior side was out. Had we qualified, we would have become absorbed in a reunified Germany and we probably would not have gone to the tournament anyway because, as of October 1990, East Germany officially no longer existed. Either way, it was no longer a problem because we weren't going anyway! If I'm honest, I would have loved to have represented my country at one last World Cup, but the reunification, while liberating and the result of people power, also meant the death knell for the majority of East Germany's international football careers, myself included.

I think Matthias Sammer was the first big name to move from East to West a few months later, and he was followed by Andreas Thom and a host of others the following summer. We were free and we could do what we wanted.

When people ask me about life in East Germany, I tell them I had a very happy childhood, the government paid everything for me, including my training and education, so I was well looked after, and that I had no real cause for complaint. But now the borders were open and we were free to do what we wanted. Many people were afraid of what came next because, not unlike prisoners who'd been in jail for most of their lives and were used to being told what to do, many were institutionalised.

I looked at the West Germany squad and I knew I was never going to be able to compete with Jurgen Klinsmann, Rudi Voller, Thomas Doll – the list was endless and, of course, they would go on and win the 1990 World Cup, so I pushed away all thoughts of playing for the reunified Germany. I was always optimistic and had belief in my own ability and a desire to succeed, but I was a realist, too. In one sense, I hoped East Germany would keep its identity, like Scotland or Wales, but still be part of the new Germany, but that was never going to happen.

## KNOCKING DOWN WALLS

I won my fifth and final cap in East Germany's last-ever game against Belgium, which was a very emotional and proud moment for all the East German players who took part. Only Matthias Sammer returned out of the big stars that had gone to play in the Bundesliga. We won the game 2-0 in Belgium and many fans made the journey to mark what was a historic occasion. We had the biggest party ever afterwards for the players and all the coaches and support staff who had been around the national team for so many years. We were paid a massive bonus for winning, because the authorities had to get rid of all the currency, but I was just glad I was there and was part of it because it was still my country. I never felt less than proud to wear that jersey.

# 6

## Verloren im Übergang

### (Lost in transition)

My first full season at Magdeburg should have ended in glory, but we blew it on the last day of the campaign. The scenario was simple: if we won our final match, we won the Oberliga. Failure wasn't an option and the title would have been the icing on the cake for what had been a wonderful year, both on a personal level and for the team. We were the surprise package – considering we'd fought relegation the season before – we just had to see ourselves over the finish line.

We were leading the league by four points at Christmas and were really firing on all cylinders, with our perfect mix of experience down the spine and younger players throughout the rest of the team. We were a sensation but I lost my strike partner, Markus Wuckel, who was badly injured in a car crash that effectively ended his season and we lost our momentum in the second half of the season. We didn't score anywhere near as many goals as we had been doing, but we were still clinging on at the top. It had become a three-horse race between Magdeburg, Dynamo Dresden and third-placed FC Karl-Marx-Stadt – Karl-Marx being our last game of the season.

We'd run out of steam a week too soon and we lost 1-0. I was emotionally and physically drained – we all were – because it had been such a crazy year. To lose the title on the final day after playing the kind of the football we'd played all season was devastating. Karl-Marx-Stadt leapfrogged us, and Dynamo Dresden, the defending champions, took the title on goal difference. I didn't turn up for the medal ceremony because I knew that had been our moment in time and we'd failed to see the job over the line. I should have done, but I just couldn't stomach it.

My manager and mentor, Joachim Streich, moved to Eintracht Braunschweig in the summer and a few of our best players left too. Things went quickly downhill thereafter.

I played for half a season but I was starting to get restless. I didn't have an agent at the time but I got to know a businessman from Bremen whose name was Hans Koziol, who had made his fortune in one-armed bandits within casinos. He would become a very good friend and advisor and, in many ways, I became the son he never had. He came from the north of West Germany and arrived at FC Magdeburg, where he was friends with Paul Seguin – a first-team co-ordinator who I was very close to and who looked after me. I ate at his house and stayed with his family when I was alone. He was a former player who only wanted good things for me.

He introduced me to Hans, who had scored the winning goal in the European Cup Final against AC Milan in the mid-1970s. I didn't have a girlfriend or wife at the time and he sort of adopted me into his family and explained that while he wasn't an agent, he could speak to other clubs on my behalf, to help take the pressure off me and sift the wheat from the chaff. He could sniff the bullshit a mile away and though he acted as my agent, that's not what he actually was.

I was being contacted by several other Bundesliga clubs and my head was spinning, but Hans was my filter; he listened to what the clubs were offering and managed to figure out who was serious and who wasn't. Ultimately, it came down to just Stuttgart and Werder Bremen, but after careful consideration, I didn't feel quite ready for life in the West so when Dynamo Dresden came in for me, in my mind it offered me the best of both worlds.

Hans negotiated three contracts but left the final decision to me, but he was happy to help me invest my new-found wealth wisely. I hadn't a clue what to do because everything I'd known was changing, including the tax system – previously there had been no tax declarations – and I desperately needed guidance to protect my future. Perhaps a little naively, I gave Hans a lot of my money to invest on my behalf and, in hindsight, things could have gone badly wrong – but they didn't. I barely knew this man, but instinctively I did trust him. He ensured every penny was accounted for and invested wisely in conservative projects such as property and, as a result, I bought a number of apartments in East Germany that I still own today. I was lucky

– many other players who were in similar situations were not and lost everything.

I could have gone crazy, splashing out money here, there and everywhere, but instead I lived a fairly normal life and whichever club I was at, I leased a car for 12 months because of the favourable rates footballers were given, and then changed it after a year. Even then I never went for anything too flashy and would get a mid-range BMW or something similar. I owed so much to Hans and remained close friends with him until his death in 2008.

Dresden paid almost two million German marks, or about £900,000 for me. It was a record fee between two East German clubs and that remained in place for about 14 years. It was a massive transfer that made me a relatively rich man at the time. Dresden were a strong club with a great tradition and they represented an opportunity for me to stay in the East, yet play in the Bundesliga. The Oberliga was to be combined with the Bundesliga but because of the strength of the West German teams, East German clubs would have to earn the right to play in one of Europe's strongest divisions. Only the teams finishing in the top two of the Oberliga were guaranteed a Bundesliga berth for the 1991/92 season, while those finishing between third and sixth would go into a play-off for the remaining places. The rest of the teams would be dispersed between 2.Bundesliga and the lower divisions and, inevitably, some would cease to exist.

Dresden's incredible history of titles and record in European competition – plus the fact they rarely finished out of the top three – made the decision to move there easier, though it was still a gamble given I'd had the opportunity to join established

Bundesliga teams. The Berlin Wall may have gone, but the new freedom took a lot of adjusting for a lot of people and maybe, looking back, I was one of them.

Like any new player coming in, I would have to prove myself worthy of wearing the shirt as well as having to justify the fee the club had paid for me. But there was the added pressure at Dresden of replacing one of the best players in Germany, let alone East Germany. Ulf Kirsten had been compared to the great Gerd Muller in that he was fairly short in height but built like a tank. He had a low centre of gravity that made him technically excellent on the ground, as well as being just as dangerous in the air.

He had signed for Bayer Leverkusen and would become the first player to win a combined 100 caps – 49 for East Germany, 51 for Germany – so I was stepping into a sizeable pair of boots. I wondered whether Dresden fans would take to me because we were two totally different players.

Things went quite well and we were there or thereabouts in the league and also progressing well in the European Cup, though I was ineligible for the next round of the competition against Malmo, which we drew 1-1 both home and away. We edged through on penalties in Sweden and our 'reward' was being drawn against favourites Red Star Belgrade in the quarter-finals, playing the first leg in Belgrade. What an occasion that was – it was the greatest atmosphere I've ever experienced in what was known as the 'Balkan Maracana', with maybe 90,000 people making a hell of a racket.

If we progressed past this round, we'd be in with a great chance of making the final, but Red Star were one of the strongest teams in the world at that time with players like Dejan

Savicevic, Darko Pancev and Robert Prosinecki, and each one could have walked into any side in the world.

We gave it our best shot but they took us apart in the first leg and were 3-0 up before we'd even played an hour, so the tie was as good as over. That said, if we were to produce something close to a miracle, we'd need a flying start in Dresden – and we got it through a Torsten Gutschow penalty after just three minutes. We defended like lions and knew that if we could sneak another goal, we'd be in with a real chance.

Our fans were frantic, willing us on and the emotions filtered down to the pitch. We held out for 50 minutes before Savicevic levelled for Belgrade and effectively killed the tie. Pancev made it 2-1 on 71 minutes and our fans had seen enough, throwing flares onto the pitch and causing mayhem in the stands. The match was abandoned after 78 minutes and UEFA awarded Belgrade a 3-0 win, so the record books say they went through in a canter, 6-0 on aggregate, but in reality it was much closer than that. The riots at Dresden meant we were banned from European competition for 12 months, too, so those disturbances cost the club dearly.

Red Star went on to beat Bayern Munich in the semi-finals and then faced Marseille in the final, drawing 0-0 but winning 5-3 on penalties, so at least we had the consolation of knowing we'd been beaten by the eventual champions.

I had joined in the January, and though I felt the supporters were initially a little reserved towards me, I think I started to win them over because I gave 100 per cent every time I played. The results were good, too, and we finished second in the Oberliga and were now officially a Bundesliga side, which was a tremendous achievement. It also meant that I would at last have the chance to fulfil my boyhood dream of playing in Germany's premier league, and we'd done it on merit, too. I was happy at Dresden and with how things were going, but the coach who had signed me, Reinhard Häfner, was sacked at the end of the season.

Dresden replaced Häfner with Helmut Schulte, who they believed had the necessary CV to help keep the club in the top division. Schulte had done a decent job with St Pauli and brought in a number of players from his native West Germany, but attracting big names to Dresden was difficult. It wasn't about the money; it was the lifestyle and dreary Communist surroundings that put perspective signings off.

I had the added problem that I wasn't his signing so I'd need to prove myself all over again. The objective for our first Bundesliga season in 1991/92 was simple – survive. Hansa Rostock was the only other East German side in that inaugural reunified Bundesliga, and they were realistic enough to have similar goals. It was a massive leap for both clubs, both on and off the pitch. We were travelling to the West as free men and there was no Stasi keeping tabs on us, no rumours of players fleeing while abroad and a million other items of mental baggage that we used to carry around with us.

I felt I'd had a good season and done myself justice, especially as I'd scored as many goals as Kirsten had that season, but I probably didn't quite reach his levels of consistency as often as I would have liked – there were very few strikers in Germany who could have matched his game. But we'd acquitted ourselves well at a far higher standard of football than we'd been used to. It hadn't been an easy transition, but we'd dug deep and ground out results when we had to.

# KNOCKING DOWN WALLS

Reunification brought many good things, but it also exposed us to the western freedom of speech in the media and suddenly the respectful straight reporting we'd been used to all our lives was replaced by tabloid sensationalism and as a record East German buy, I found myself constantly in the spotlight. It seemed to happen overnight and it seemed I couldn't move without attracting the attention of a photographer or a snooping journalist. It would take some getting used to and being only 22, I was nowhere near ready for the intensive scrutiny, gossip and tittle-tattle of my professional and personal life.

Being under the microscope began to weigh as heavily on my shoulders as the record transfer fee. I was young for my age and the pressure was beginning to affect my game, but I felt I was learning fast and adapting my style accordingly. We often had our backs to the wall in matches and were trying to also play the style our new manager wanted. As a result, the goals would prove harder to come by.

I needed a strong first season to prove I could cut it in the Bundesliga and we started our adventure knowing we were going to have to scrap for every point and that there would be, pardon the cliché, no easy games. In many ways it was like coming from the Championship in England into the Premier League, and every game was a cup final. We knew that West German teams wouldn't be comfortable coming to Dresden, which was still exactly the same as it had been under the Communist government and would be for several years – change of that magnitude didn't happen overnight. We had to use that to our advantage and make our home ground a fortress, so our visitors felt they were well outside their comfort zone. Just as away games were strange for us, it could work both ways.

We were travelling to big, Olympic stadiums with massive crowds and it was a whole new world for us. Sometimes we felt like spectators watching the match rather than actually competing in it, and I think some of the results back that theory up. We were overwhelmed at times, playing teams and players that previously we'd only seen on TV, and sometimes we let the occasion get the better of us.

We'd also have other factors against us in the early days, with six or seven-hour coach journeys the day before a game, which meant we were leggy and stiff at the start of some matches. It was a steep learning curve to say the least.

Dresden had no major stars and relied on team spirit and hard work to carry us through games. While this sometimes worked, more often than not it wasn't enough. The club was hemorrhaging money because the system in the East still had a long way to catch up and, financially, it was disastrous. A number of East German clubs found they could no longer operate within a very short space of time.

We still had a number of former internationals in our team and their experience – and occasionally luck – carried us through the season. There was also the odd time when we were so wound up that we dug deep to stuff the words down our detractors' throats. We were always regarded as inferior and looked down upon because we came from the East, and I recall playing Bayern Munich away from home when the opposition slurs backfired on them. Our fans had travelled in numbers because a visit to the West was still something of a novelty and a day out in Munich, a few beers and a football match appealed to many Dresden fans, with maybe 4,000 following us south.

On one occasion, I was up against a guy I had a lot of respect for – a World Cup winner in fact – and years later, I'm still willing to give him the benefit of the doubt and believe things were said in the heat of the moment. Only he knows the truth and I'm not going to name him here. He was in my ear throughout the game and verbally there were many exchanges during the game. He was trying to wind me up, maybe knowing that I had a reputation of seeing red a few years back and he said: "You East Germans, you should piss off back to where you came from. I earn more in a week than you do in a year."

We knew they looked down on us but it didn't matter where you came from, when the referee started the game it was 11 versus 11, and on this occasion we taught Munich a lesson and beat them 2-1. I gave a wink to the guy who'd suggested we didn't belong in the Bundesliga, shook his hand and that was the end of that, but it was not uncommon during that season.

Dresden's style was not helping my game and I was just about holding my own in the team. The passing style was completely different from Magdeburg, who were very much a counter-attacking team who played with width and wingers and I've always played my best football in that system. Dresden played a short, narrow passing game and everything was through the middle. Whereas before I'd been bursting into the box to get on the end of crosses, here I played with my back to goal more often than not, holding the ball up and looking for the odd threaded pass. I tried to adjust my game but I don't think the fans ever really took to me. Only our situation and the 'us v them' mentality helped my cause, because we were all in it together and no matter what, the fans backed me and the team.

It was hard for our coaches, too, because they, like us, had only known the Oberliga, so in order to survive, many clubs drafted in West German coaches, believing they would have the experience and knowledge to succeed and understand better the kind of players that were best suited to the challenge ahead. It meant many East German coaches had nowhere to go and there were many players, too, who were lost in the transition and forced to play or work at a much lower standard.

Our home and away form could not have been more different. Away we were distracted and, at times, all over the place defensively, suffering a number of heavy defeats, but at home we were focused and a completely different proposition. We shipped very few goals and kept maybe 10 clean sheets out of 18 home games, gathering most of our points in Dresden in front of regular crowds of 30,000.

We felt like we were representing our part of the country in that first season and I believe all the fans from every club supported ourselves and Hansa Rostock – if we failed, what would that say about the standard of East German football as a whole? We were carrying more than the hopes and dreams of our own supporters; we were playing for our country's pride.

By the end of the season, we avoided relegation by three points, but Hansa Rostock were relegated. It was not far off a sensation that we had survived because we had been dismissed as no-hopers and were favourites for relegation before a ball had even been kicked. I don't know if people had any respect for us when we began the season, but I'm certain they did by the end. It was a fascinating year, not the most productive on a personal level, but I was certainly part of a team who many had written off as little more than amateurs.

With another season in the Bundesliga guaranteed, I had to figure out whether my future lay elsewhere. That first full year had been an adventure and we'd been set the challenge of proving we were up to the task, but having achieved that, the prospect of another relegation battle didn't excite me. The style of football showed no sign of changing and the supporters, I felt, may not have been so lenient with me if I continued to struggle to find the net, as I had done in that first Bundesliga season. If an interesting option presented itself, I decided I would take it on, whether in the West or the East.

There was a problem with my relationship with Helmut Schulte, in that there wasn't one. I wouldn't say we didn't get along, but it wasn't productive. He hadn't signed me, I wasn't his sort of player and in the end we didn't see eye to eye on virtually anything. Add to that the fact I'd scored just nine goals in 51 appearances and we agreed to disagree. In a situation like that, moving on is inevitable.

I felt ready for something different and so when FC Nürnberg, an established Bundesliga side from Bavaria, came in for me I was happy to move, even though I felt a strong bond with Dresden after the shared experience of promotion and that first Bundesliga campaign. Nürnberg paid 1.2m German marks for me – about £700,000 – which was still big money. But it meant I moved out of the East for the first time in my life, though it would be a decision I would regret for the rest of my career...

## 1

# Eine Katastrophe nach der anderen

## (One disaster after another)

Things began okay for me at Nürnberg and I started every game, as you'd expect of such an expensive signing. However, as had happened in the past, I shot myself in the foot at a relatively early stage of my career there, and that set the tone for my time with the club.

A month or so into my spell there, I saw red again during a match, losing my head and being given my marching orders. I was banned for eight games, so I'd pissed off the manager and the supporters straight away by doing something stupid. Worse still, I hadn't managed to score for them in the Bundesliga up to that point, so there were still plenty of question marks in people's minds about whether I was actually worth the money that had been spent on me.

I was up against it and, as the only East German in the team, I was hardly embraced by my team-mates and felt on the outside. Their culture was alien to me and I found it difficult to integrate myself because there were too many cliques within the squad.

I'd been brought up to believe that everyone pulled together and, no matter what your age or status, you were part of a team. At FC Nürnberg, there were a number of experienced players who called a lot of the shots. One or two seemed to train only when they felt like it and one senior pro, Hans Dorfner, a former West German international, appeared to have, in my opinion, way too much influence at the club – sometimes it even felt as though he was picking the team on occasions!

I'm not saying Willi Entenmann, the coach, was weak – but he was certainly influenced by Dorfner and I clearly wasn't his cup of tea. Dorfner was a powerful character in the dressing room and, don't get me wrong, a great player, but he was at the wrong end of his career, very injury prone and, in my opinion, he was having a negative effect on the club.

I wasn't exactly frozen out by my team-mates and I had some friends among the squad, but it was also true that I wasn't welcomed with open arms, either. It worked both ways and I know now I didn't go out of my way to integrate myself into the squad. My failure to settle in and my lack of goals and early suspension meant that I was miserable and lonely. Every chance I had, I returned home to Leipzig – another mistake. I should have tried to immerse myself more into Nürnberg life and discovered what made the city tick and what was important to the club's supporters; instead, I was treating it as somewhere I worked but didn't live.

I started to question myself, too. Did I miss the way things were before reunification? Could I adjust and move on? The Berlin Wall may have gone forever, but for many people it still existed and there was still a West Germany and an East Germany in many respects. A mental divide still existed and it was equally as powerful as the physical blockade that had split the nation in two.

The fact I could jump in the car and be where I considered home was proving more of a negative than a positive. In Leipzig, I would relax, socialise and be with my friends – until I had to return to Nürnberg, where I continued to feel like an outcast and was increasingly distancing myself from the club.

I only went home on my day off or the day after the game, but when I did, I often trained with my old club Chemie Leipzig – and my employers were totally unaware of this. There was no Internet back then to spread rumours, no mobile phone pictures or social media and there were no photographers camped outside Chemie's training ground, so that was how I handled my home sickness.

I attended every Nürnberg training session, too, but the trips home, the training with Chemie and my failure to settle suggested I wasn't moving on with my life as I had intended. My career was suffering too because I had scored just seven Bundesliga goals in almost two years.

I did make a couple of friends – pals who I still have to this day in the shape of Andreas Kopke, who is now the goalkeeping coach for the national team, and striker Dieter Eckstein.

I returned to the team and found the net in a couple of cup matches, but I still couldn't end my goal drought in the league and it was destroying me. The longer it went on, the more anxiety crept into my game and I was missing chances I would normally score with my eyes closed – there was no end to it.

Entenmann never dropped me though, which suggests goals were perhaps the only thing missing from my game. I worked hard and contributed to the team but, as a striker, your goals column is king. I was disappointed, then, to be relegated to the bench for the final game of the season. I had gone 28 games without a Bundesliga goal and, though my pride was hurting, I couldn't really question the manager's decision.

Then came the moment that told me my time with Nürnberg was at an end. Midway through the second half, the boss told me to get stripped off and I walked to the touchline ready to come on. The Nürnberg fans applauded the guy coming off and then I ran on to the pitch after we'd given each other a high five – and the whole stadium booed. I was finished. It was horrible and something I would never forget. It capped off a terrible year for me.

Yet, there was to be a silver lining and something that literally came out of the blue. Despite my unpopularity and lack of goals, I received a call-up for a training camp for the national team – something I thought would never happen, particularly after I'd just bombed at Nürnberg! The news couldn't have come at a better time because I was on my knees confidence-wise and, yet, Berti Vogts, the national coach, had seen something in my game that he liked. Okay, it wasn't the first 15 I would be joining – more the players ranked 16 to 30 – but, for me, it didn't matter. It meant I was in the mind of the national coach and on the fringes of the team who were the world champions. Maybe I wasn't such a bad player after all!

I attended the training camp feeling a massive weight had been lifted off my shoulders. So, I joined the group at a Sportschule in Duisburg and, of course, I scored in the internal match we played behind closed doors. There was plenty of Bundesliga talent there and I did more than okay on the day.

In the meantime, Ralf Minge, a former team-mate of mine, was appointed caretaker-coach at Dynamo Dresden at the end of the season, and he made it clear that he wanted me to return. Minge was confident of landing the job on a permanent basis – he knew my game inside out and he sold the move to me. Nürnberg agreed it was best I didn't return for another season after the way the previous campaign had ended, and allowed me to move on a season-long loan deal to Dresden. It was exactly what I needed and I thought I could return home, rediscover my form and then venture out having learned my lessons. For me, it was a win-win situation.

However, Minge wasn't given the job [although he stayed on as assistant-manager], and Siggi Held was appointed instead. Not for the first time I would again be a player someone else had brought in. Plus, there was a catch. Unbeknown to me, Dresden and Nürnberg had struck a deal that, had I been aware of, I would never have agreed to the move.

Dresden would pay my wages and there would be no fee for my 12-month loan. However, each time I played before the 75th minute, Dresden would have to pay a fee of 5,000DM, which was a lot of money, particularly for a club like Dresden, who were in serious financial difficulty.

The season started and Dresden were forced to begin with a four-point deduction for financial irregularities, so it wasn't an ideal beginning to the campaign – but, for me, things were about to get even worse.

## KNOCKING DOWN WALLS

I played the first six Bundesliga games and failed to end my scoring drought, which now stretched to more than 40 games, but my career in East German football was about to come to a shuddering end after I went up for a header and came down awkwardly, collapsing in pain on the floor immediately aware I'd done something seriously wrong.

My ankle blew up like a balloon, and subsequent x-rays and scans later confirmed that my ankle ligaments had completely detached from the bone. I would require an operation to repair the damage.

To compound my fortunes, in my absence, Dresden went on a really good run which was great for the club, but not so good for my prospects of a permanent deal. By January, I had worked my way back to fitness, but it was clear my time with Dresden was over. The coach told me the team had done very well without me, the strikers were scoring goals and that it would be better for all parties if I moved on – how could I disagree?

I decided that was enough and that I needed to leave Germany completely because whatever it was that was holding me back showed no sign of releasing its grip. I felt I was under some kind of curse.

So, where next? Wherever I decided to go, it had to be right. I needed a completely fresh start and that got me thinking about a time when I was still making my way through the youth ranks at Lokomotive Leipzig. Back when I shared a room with Mathias and Ingo at the school of excellence, I recalled one of the lads had an old C60 tape which we played constantly. It had English football fans singing many different songs – 'You'll Never Walk Alone', 'We're On the March', 'We Shall Not Be Moved' and many, many others – probably taped off a radio during coverage of English matches. We all loved English football, the passion of the fans, the tradition and the stadiums and we used to talk about what it would be like to play in front of supporters like that. I made my mind up to follow my instincts and look to move to the English Premiership, to effectively relaunch my career – it just felt right on a number of levels.

The guy who had helped me move from Nürnberg to Dresden felt bad that things had not worked out for me and also that I'd been kept in the dark regarding certain aspects of the deal. He wanted to put things right with me, so I said: "Okay, find me a club in England."

He was as good as his word and introduced me to Wolfgang Vöge, who was – and still is – one of the biggest football agents in Europe.

Wolfgang had fantastic connections all over the place and for some reason, considering he also counted some of the biggest names in world football as his clients, he seemed to take a real shine to me and took me under his wing.

I spoke with him and we agreed that the best option was to go abroad, rebuild and then return a more complete player and a more rounded individual. I told him I'd always wanted to go to England and he said: "Okay, why not?"

There was something different about English football that really appealed to me, so, when Wolfgang arranged a trial for me at Middlesbrough, it seemed like the perfect chance for me to follow my dream. I flew to Teesside Airport, stayed in a hotel in Stockton and watched Oldham Athletic playing live on TV that evening. The next day, I was picked up by a club driver and, although I'd been told I would be training with the first-team, they weren't around, so I actually did a little workout with the reserves. It wasn't anything too strenuous, so I was less than impressed.

The following day, I was meant to be playing in a reserve game, but that was called off due to heavy snowfall. It had been, thus far, a complete waste of time.

I flew back to Germany the day after that and once again wondered if I was travelling under some sort of jinx. However, I'd no sooner landed than I got another call from Wolfgang, who told me he'd arranged a trial at Manchester City. I was to fly to Manchester the following Monday, where I would be training with the first-team and then playing in a reserve game against Burnley on the Tuesday evening. After the Middlesbrough experience, I didn't get too excited, but I knew that Manchester City were a much bigger club and hoped that, for once, fate was smiling on me.

I'd been out for almost six months and was nowhere near fit enough for the reserve game against Burnley, but I gave it my all, scored twice and, by the 55th minute, I had cramp and was exhausted because I hadn't played competitively for so long. God bless first-team manager Brian Horton for taking me off when he did, as I think things would have deteriorated rapidly after that. It felt good to know I could still score goals and I was happy enough with my display.

I took a shower and went up to meet Brian in the boardroom after the match had finished. He told me he was pleased with what he'd seen and that he was taking me on until the end of the season. I was also going to be included in the squad to face QPR at Loftus Road the following Saturday.

Things had gone so smoothly that I was waiting for something bad to happen, such was my mind-set at the time. However, it didn't, and the dreams I'd had since I was a kid were all about to come true. After a lot of wandering and restlessness, I was struck immediately by an overwhelming feeling that I'd finally found what I was looking for.

# Endlich zu Hause

## (Home at last)

All the financial aspects had been agreed with Nürnberg and I trained with the rest of the lads a couple of times before making my debut against QPR. City were fourth-from-bottom of the Premiership and in trouble. They had won just two of their last 20 league games, so we needed points and quickly.

I made my debut at Loftus Road and I remember running out for the first time for a top flight English league game. It was a great feeling to see the supporters in the stands and at QPR, the crowd is right on top of you – there was no running track around the pitch, so you could hear comments from individuals, though my English was thankfully poor at that time! The sun was shining and I was raring to go, but my fitness was still lacking, somewhat. I'd put a lot into the reserve game in midweek and tried to impress during the training sessions, so I was feeling a little jaded going into the match. But I had enough energy to get down the flank, whip a cross in and David Rocastle timed his run to perfection to plant the ball home. We drew 1-1 and it was a useful point under the circumstances.

I needed to get my match fitness up to scratch as soon as possible, but I had a number of obstacles to get over, too. As I say, my English was pretty much non-existent and nobody really spoke any German, so there were a lot of hand gestures and pointing in the early training sessions and more than one misunderstanding. We had been taught English at school, but only very basic stuff and the teacher wasn't very good – there was no real purpose to learn English in East Germany because we'd never use it and it was treated as something that seemed fairly pointless, like learning Latin, whereas I'd had 10 years or so of being taught Russian.

I didn't understand anything that was being said apart from the odd word here and there; certainly nowhere near enough to hold a conversation, so that was something I needed to sort pretty quickly. But I was lucky in that I was coming into a team that had a lot of experience with players such as Steve McMahon, Tony Coton, Keith Curle and Niall Quinn. McMahon was a great help in those early months by taking me to one side and explaining things to me when needed. He told me what to do and what not to do in English football, and it helped me settle in a lot quicker. I really appreciated him taking the time to do that because he didn't have to.

During the next few weeks, City signed Paul Walsh from Portsmouth and Peter Beagrie from Everton before the transfer deadline as Horton re-shaped his forward line. Both Walshy and Beags would become lifelong friends in later years and we all hit it off pretty much straight away, which would soon show when we played together. Steffen Karl also arrived which made things a bit easier for me because I could speak to someone in my own language. He was also East German and had come through the youth system in a similar way I had. I'd also played against him a few times. He had joined Borussia Dortmund and made a really promising start to his career, but he had one or two off-field problems that started to affect his progress.

He was a good kid but he perhaps enjoyed the nightlife more than he should have done. He had a sharp tongue and maybe spoke before he thought on occasions, so was naïve in that respect, but he had enormous potential. I felt City played him in the wrong position. He was not a right-winger, more a central midfielder but he never had the opportunity to play there, so I don't think we ever saw the best of him.

The new signings seemed to give the club and supporters a boost at just the right time because prior to our arrival, the team had seemingly been heading for relegation. We had, in effect, a new forward line and it was like a breath of fresh air to a team that had been going stale and who seemingly lacked imagination up front.

I was staying at the Copthorne Hotel in Salford Quays, as was David Rocastle and Steffen Karl for the first few months, as we all settled into Manchester life. 'Rocky' was a great guy, very kind and good company and I had a lot of time for him. In years to come he would be taken from us long before his time due to cancer, which was a genuine tragedy. I feel privileged to have been able to play alongside him briefly and to have called him a friend.

All the players made me feel at home and went out of their way to help me in any way they could. If they went out to lunch, they always invited me to come along and I was on the golf course with them whenever there was a game going, all of which helped my English improve at a fairly rapid rate. The camaraderie reminded me a lot of my early days in East German football at Chemie Leipzig and Magdeburg, where we did everything together as a team.

Back on the pitch my home debut didn't go too well as we lost 1-0 to Wimbledon before drawing our next three games. In those first few games alongside Walshy, things didn't go too well as we couldn't communicate at all during matches. We weren't operating as a partnership and we'd run in the same channels on occasion, leave it to each other at other times and it was a little embarrassing, but we were both willing each other to do well and trying our best for the team.

I recall one time when we both chased a long ball and we collided as we approached the ball – it was a nightmare and we had a joke about it after the game over a beer. We weren't scoring and in those first few weeks, we didn't look like we were going to hit it off as a pair. After a 0-0 draw with Sheffield United, Walshy stopped at a motorway services to grab something to eat and he was confronted by a busload of Man United fans who started singing: 'What an impact you have made! What an impact you have made!' He just had to eat his sandwich and let them get on with it as he had no comeback at that point.

But with each passing game, we were starting to understand how each other worked and improving. The goals still didn't come as we drew 0-0 at Oldham Athletic, but the movement was better and with Beags adding another dimension to our attack with his superb wing play and crosses, we started to gel.

Finally, away to Ipswich Town, I scored my first goal and, even better, Walshy scored, too, so we both ended our barren run in the same game. We drew 2-2 but we were off and running and it was as though a huge weight had been lifted and things improved at a rapid rate from then on. I scored my first goal at Maine Road in the next game, as did Walshy, and Beags added another as we beat Aston Villa 3-0, meaning we'd lost just once in the past eight games. Everything had suddenly clicked. From bumping into each other during games and, at times, looking like we would never forge an effective partnership, it had all clicked into place.

Sometimes, as I've learned over the years, it never happens and two players can be like chalk and cheese, but we couldn't afford to fail. It was vital for the club and for my future in English football that it finally had. Our confidence shot up and it wasn't as important that we communicated verbally anymore as we understood each other on a football level, which was all that we needed.

With McMahon and Rocastle in midfield, we had experience and guile behind us and Beags was proving to be an excellent signing by Horton. His crossing was among the best I'd come across in my playing career and we survived comfortably in the end, with my goal on the last day away to Sheffield Wednesday meaning I'd scored five in 12 matches, which was a decent return given my drought at Nürnberg. I'd come to City – a struggling side – at a fairly low point in my career with my confidence and fitness nowhere near the levels I'd enjoyed a few seasons before, so I was elated by the way things had gone. I felt at home and really happy and I knew this was where I wanted to be next season. Better still, we had 5,000 fans for our last game at Hillsborough and we were well clear of the relegation zone.

After my goal, the City fans began to sing my name to the tune of 'Go West' and it went on throughout the match. I'd never heard my name sung before and initially, because I was so focused on the game, I didn't realise they were singing about me or what they were singing. Back home, supporters had maybe one song for the whole club and didn't sing about individual players, so it was all new to me. But it went on and on and when I finally realised it was my name that was echoing around this famous old English stadium, it made the hairs stand up on the back of neck. All those years ago, as a kid, I'd listened on a tape to English songs being sung and now here I was and it was happening to me. It didn't get much better than that and though I'd had a relationship with the fans of the majority of teams I'd played for, I'd never had anything like this before. As we made our way home along the Snake Pass back to Manchester, we were followed by a mass convey of supporters behind us and I suppose I just fell in love with the club, the fans and England.

With the season over, I wanted the loan deal made permanent as quickly as possible, but was surprised when my agent told me that Sheffield Wednesday had also put in a bid for me – offering me more money, too – probably based on my performance against them. Trevor Francis was the manager and he was really keen for me to join and I was advised that, on paper, it was a better deal. But I wasn't interested in money after the past two years of feeling that I'd stood still, I really wanted to kick on. I told my agent I wanted to stay at City where I felt appreciated, was happy with the players around me and the area and the contract offer was decent, too. I had no intention of going anywhere else and was already looking forward to starting the new season as a Manchester City player.

Besides, I had already formed a close relationship with the manager, Brian Horton, his coaching staff and first-team coach Tony Book, who I spent a lot of time with off the field and who I grew very fond of.

City paid £375,000 for me and because I was the first German to play football in England for a number of years, I knew there were a lot of eyes on me both here and back in Germany. It was not like it had been in Bert Trautmann's day, of course, but I still felt I had to win over the general public because the relationship between our two countries was still one of suspicion. Francis Lee was a clever man and I think he got a great deal paying what he did. I think he saw Germany as an area he could buy quality at a bargain price, at least with some players, and the Bundesliga was an area he would re-visit a number of times during his reign as City chairman.

As for Steffen Karl, like me, he joined City on loan with a view to a permanent deal, but he only made a handful of appearances and returned to Germany after the season ended. There were a number of reasons things didn't work out for him and he probably realised in later years they were mostly of his own making.

Towards the end of the season, we went on a trip to the Channel Islands and I remember Brian Horton got everyone together after the meal we'd had at the hotel and Steffen said: "Hey gaffer, maybe it's time to send the kids to bed now?" Everybody just looked at him, especially as he was one of the youngest in the travelling party, but it was typical Steffen, not engaging his brain before talking. I don't think Brian fancied him as a player or a person and after we were beaten 2-0 at Man United just before the end of the season, he was substituted early into the second half. He went straight to the changing rooms, got changed and disappeared. After the game, I was in the dressing room and where Steffen had sat, there was a piece of white tape with a message written in German. The gaffer asked me where he was and I told him I didn't know, but I knew the message read: 'Pick me up from the Copthorne Hotel. I'll be in the bar.'

Unfortunately for Steffen, there was a get-together planned after the match with all the players, manager and Francis Lee attending – at the Copthorne Hotel – and when we arrived there, he was at the bar with a whisky and coke. I think that was pretty much the end for him at City.

Our last home game the season was against Chelsea and it was also the final match to be played in front of the Kippax terrace, which I'd grown to love in a very short space of time. The atmosphere inside English grounds was exactly as I had imagined it would be all those years ago and I knew I was in the perfect place. I loved playing in front of the Kippax and feel privileged that I had the chance to play in front of the City fans who would create such a great atmosphere. I may have only had six games in front of the old Kippax, but the memories I have are very special and things weren't quite the same after the new, all-seater Kippax was built.

Back home, the Press had picked up on my progress with City and I was reading good, positive things. English football was popular in Germany and the fact that I was now the only German playing here made me feel good about myself. It had been the right decision to leave the Bundesliga behind, though it was always in my mind that maybe one day I'd have another crack at it. I had a good summer back at Leipzig with my friends and family and prepared well for the 1994/95 season, which I hoped to hit the ground running. I was hungry again and felt in a very good place, so when I came back for pre-season, I was in the best possible state to begin my first full season in England.

It was hard, too. Every other day we had running, running and more running and I was soon in good shape for what lay ahead. I couldn't have been any happier and the pre-season trip to Norway would also bring an unexpected bonus that would have a massive impact on my life and my future. We went for around 10 days and split our base between Horten and Oslo while we played our games. At our hotel, the Grand Ocean, I met a girl who I had no idea would one day become my wife and mother of my two sons. She was working as a receptionist and we got talking one day, which wasn't easy as I was still learning English and she spoke no German.

I was in my mid-twenties and had no previous girlfriends, certainly no long-term relationships as such. I suppose I was ready for some stability in my personal life, too, so to meet Cecilie when I did was perfect timing. One thing I felt that was missing from my life was a companion and I knew that to be settled on the pitch, I needed to be settled off it. Coming back to an empty flat after a great game would be a grounding, lonely experience and I suppose I was looking to meet the right girl and maybe start a family. I guess the moment I first saw her I knew she was the one.

We arranged an evening out and my team-mate, Michel Vonk, offered to interpret for us because he knew a little German and his English was good, as was Cecilie's, but it obviously wasn't ideal! Vonk told her what I wanted to say – I hope so, anyway! I have no idea what he was telling her but we exchanged numbers and began to phone each other but as you can imagine, it wasn't easy.

On the last day of the tour, Brian gave us the night off in Oslo and I met up with Cecilie. We managed to have a good time despite the communication problems. I discovered she was studying business and had saved to take a one-year course in Sydney, Australia, where she would take a course in business. The hotel job was just a means to save enough money for the trip which was already paid for and booked. She came over to stay with me at my apartment in Bramhall for Christmas before she started her course in Australia.

We continued to keep in touch and even though she was now on the other side of the world and our conversations were limited to say the least, we were finding it harder and harder to stay apart. Then she decided things weren't going the way she'd planned and managed to transfer her course to London.

She left the sun, sea and lifestyle so we could see each other more, even though we hardly knew each other in reality. As it turned out, good accommodation in London was hard to find, so I offered her the option of moving in with me, which she did while still commuting to her course in London. It was quite a commitment from her and it was the start of our life together.

# 9

# Treten auf

## (Kicking on)

One thing I've done at a number of clubs is start the season off on a bad note, and I was furious at myself for it happening in the opening game of the new campaign with City. Now officially a City player, things couldn't have begun much worse as my two yellow cards resulted in a sending off away to Arsenal. My language was clearly improving as the second caution was for swearing at the referee – maybe I'd have got away with it if I hadn't picked up some of the local Moss Side lingo so quickly.

We lost 3-0 and I thought, 'here we go again.' I'd stepped over the line, trying too hard and ended up with an early bath. I thought I would be banned for six weeks as a result – just as I had been in Germany several times before. It was unthinkable that I would be out for two months and it could ruin my hopes of really establishing myself in England.

Thankfully that's not how the Premiership worked and the ban, just one match, wouldn't come into effect for another couple of games. It was a relief because I'd been determined to start the season with a real impact and it meant I was still available for the upcoming home games against West Ham United and Everton.

It was strange at Maine Road, where we now had only three stands with the Kippax demolished and the majority of our louder fans re-housed in the North Stand. It also meant our capacity was reduced to around 20,000, but it gave the home games a different feel, almost like a cup tie at another ground with a large away following behind us.

We won the first two home games 3-0 and 4-0 and I scored three goals, which was as much as I could have hoped for. As an attacking force, at times we looked like title contenders at home, but our form on the road was pretty abysmal. I must admit I also had concerns over my place in the team now Niall Quinn was fit again.

When I'd first arrived I had no idea of the status of various individuals at the club and the kind of sway they had both on and off the pitch, but after almost six months in Manchester, I was aware of what Quinny meant to City. My English was continually getting better but there was no doubt Niall was the main guy at the club. He was a great person, too; very respectful and polite and clearly someone Brian Horton had a lot of respect for, as did I. He'd been out for several months with a cruciate ligament injury and Walshy and myself had arrived at City as a direct result of his absence, so it would be interesting to see who the gaffer went with now he was fit – and he'd done really well for a big guy to get back playing as quickly as he had.

Paul Walsh and I had struck up a very good partnership that had continued through pre-season and into the new campaign. With Nicky Summerbee now on the right-wing and Beagrie on the left, we were getting fantastic service and really flying – plus we had plenty of energy with youngsters Garry Flitcroft and Steve Lomas in midfield – but the question was how Quinny would be worked into the equation? Horton's solution was that he played all of us!

The goals were flying in and I was scoring regularly, but that was because of the players I had around me. I operated best when I had good players around me and City were the right club at the right time for me to be at. My confidence was as high as it had ever been in my career and with the goals going in and the fans behind me, every time I walked out to play at Maine Road I felt unbeatable, that I could try anything and the support would be unwavering. It wasn't arrogance, just a great feeling that nothing bad would happen, whatever the circumstances. As a footballer, there's no better feeling.

I could feel the love as soon as I arrived at Maine Road and started signing autographs on the way into the ground – it was because of that feeling of being wanted that I was playing the best football of my career. It wasn't just me. Paul Walsh was scoring goals, too, and it is unusual that both players in a productive partnership be scoring goals at the same time. Normally, one suffers while the other one profits – it's just the way things go – but we were both finding the net and we were both at the top of our game. Beags was enjoying himself and you could guarantee he'd make two or three scoring chances each game, while Summerbee was playing a lot better than anyone gave him credit for. It was hard for Nicky to step out of his dad's shadow, but I thought he had a great season.

Horton had a problem though – he had wanted options, but now he had too many! Niall was a true gentleman, very complimentary and supportive and totally unselfish in every aspect of his personality. He was never jealous and he was confident in his own ability, to the point that he knew that if things didn't work out for him at City, he could pick and choose where he played. He was a fantastic player and eventually he would reclaim his place in the starting line-up. Though he initially had to make do with the subs' bench as he gradually played his way back to match fitness, on occasion we played with three up front plus the two wingers – but only at home. It was risky, but when it went well, we were devastating.

Things were going too well and I felt it couldn't possibly last. Then, against Norwich City at Maine Road, I was brought down in the box by Mike Milligan, who clattered into me. Although we won a penalty, my ankle ligaments were ruptured and I was ruled out for eight weeks. Typical! Out for the best part of a quarter of the season.

I thought that with Quinny back in the team, I would struggle to win my place back. Worse still, I missed a game I would have done anything to have played in for a number of reasons. The home match against Tottenham Hotspur was an incredible game, one of the best I've ever seen – and I had to watch it from the stand. My parents had arranged to fly over for the first time well in advance, as I would have been up against Jurgen Klinsmann, who had joined Spurs the previous summer. There was huge interest in Germany building up to the game as two

Germans would have been going head-to-head for the first time with two English clubs. It was torture.

It was also the first time I'd met Klinsmann in person and the game proved to be an absolute classic – we beat Spurs 5-2 with some scintillating football, and I was both thrilled and gutted at the same time. It's just the way things go sometimes but at least Klinsmann's arrival perhaps made people sit up and notice my form back home in Germany because before that, I think there was a more cynical approach that if I was scoring goals, the Premiership mustn't have been up to that much. But Klinsmann had such an aura that he was virtually untouchable back home. Maybe English football wasn't so bad after all?

Another good thing was that Jurgen was telling the Germany coach very complimentary things about me and I was suddenly back on the radar of the national team – all I had to do was get fit again and start scoring some more goals.

I worked very hard to get back as quickly as I could – probably too hard – but I was convinced the longer Quinny was playing and I wasn't, the harder it would be for me to win back my place. I had a minor setback during my rehab that cost me another two weeks, but after nine games out, I was back on the bench and champing at the bit to play again. I got my chance against Wimbledon at Maine Road, coming off the bench and scoring in a 2-0 win, and I came on as sub in the next game, a League Cup tie against Newcastle and scored again, so I'd sent a message to the manager and done enough to win a place in the starting XI.

Maurizio Gaudino, another German, had joined us on loan and played in the match with Newcastle. He was a talented midfielder who'd had problems at Eintracht Frankfurt. Along with Jay-Jay Okocha and Tony Yeboah, they'd been fired for reasons I'm not entirely sure of – I think they all fell out with coach Jupp Heynckes – so they all had to find new clubs. All three would come to England and make a real impact – Okocha went to Bolton, Yeboah to Leeds and Maurizio came to us.

He was a fantastic player but there was a lot of negativity surrounding him in Germany. I never asked what the problems were because I'm sure that's what he was keen to get away from so he could concentrate on his football again. I quickly discovered what a great guy he was and he settled in quickly at the club and to English life, and he really enjoyed himself here along with his wife. He also became quite close friends with Keith Curle. He had so much ability and the City fans loved him. I hoped the deal would become permanent.

So I'd won my place back for the game against Ipswich Town and I scored my third goal in three games as we won 2-1 at Portman Road to move into sixth. We were flying and I couldn't have been any happier. Plus, the German press were taking a great interest in my progress and it wasn't just a case of Klinsmann playing at Spurs, they were now writing about Uwe Rosler at Manchester City as well. I'd be lying if I didn't admit I was thrilled that I was finally getting some recognition from back home.

I'd scored 10 goals by the New Year but our form dipped after Christmas and we began to lose sight of the top-six finish we all felt we could – and should – have achieved. I did score four goals against Notts County in an FA Cup tie though, and by the end of the campaign, I'd scored 22 goals from 35 starts. I honestly believe that if I'd not been out for two months, I would have hit the 30-goal mark which, at the time, no City striker had managed since Francis Lee back in 1972.

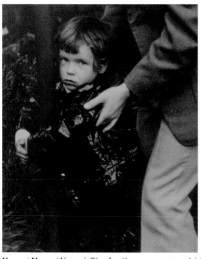

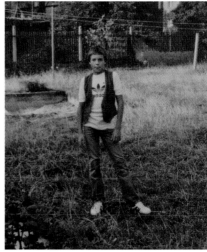

**Young Uwe:** (Above) Shy for the camera, and (right) looking trendy in my waistcoat!

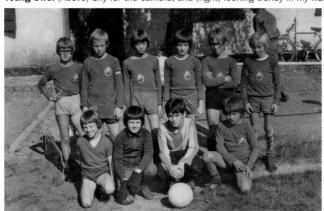

**Where it all began:** On the front row, far right, with my village side, Starkenburg

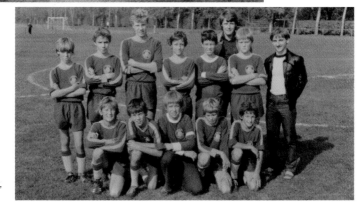

**Champions:** Lok Leipzig Under-13s, with me on the front row, second left

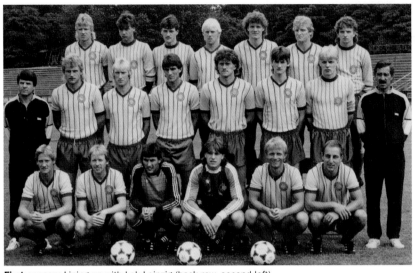

**First season:** Lining up with Lok Leipzig (back row, second left) ahead of the 1987/88 season, my first as a professional

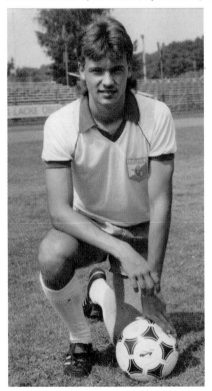

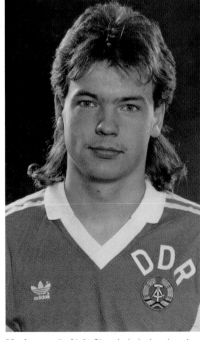

**Moving on:** (Left) At Chemie Leipzig, ahead of the 1988/89 season, and (above) in East Germany colours, for whom I won five caps

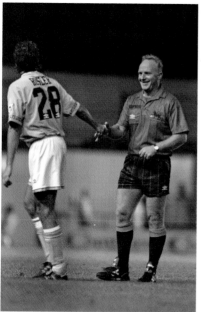

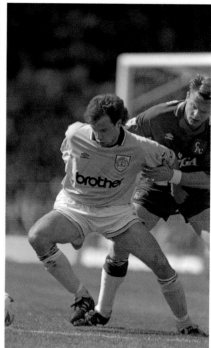

**Fair play:** Shaking hands with the referee, and (right) shielding the ball from Chelsea's Jacob Kjeldbjerg during a 2-2 draw, April 1994

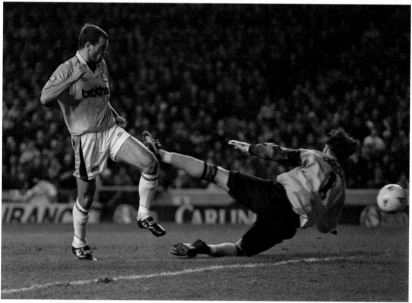

**Forest fire:** Converting from close range beyond Nottingham Forest goalkeeper Mark Crossley, during a 1-1 draw at Maine Road in December 1995

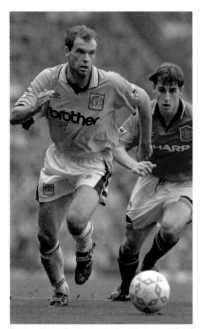
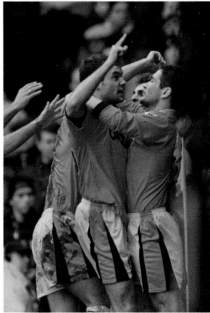

**Derby days:** On the attack with a youthful Gary Neville for company at Old Trafford, October 1995; (above right) mobbed after my goal in the FA Cup at the same venue, February 1996

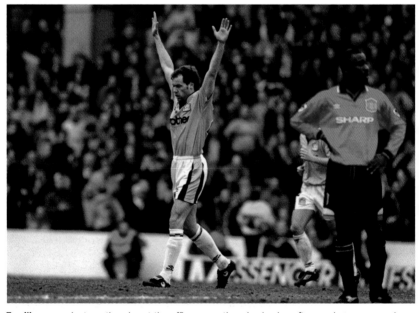

**Familiar pose:** Just another day at the office – emotions in check – after scoring our second equaliser during the Maine Road league return, April 1996

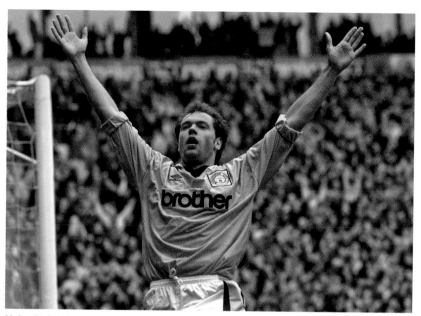

**Maine Relief:** Celebrations after scoring the only goal against Sheffield Wednesday in April 1996, our first victory in five games – surely the great escape was in sight?

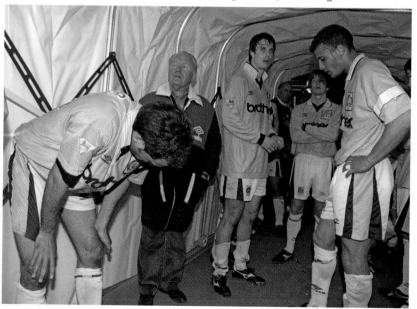

**Down and out:** In the tunnel after we'd been relegated following a 2-2 draw with Liverpool. It hadn't quite sunk in, as the faces of Kit Symons, Keith Curle and Ian Brightwell show (plus groundsman Stan Gibson)

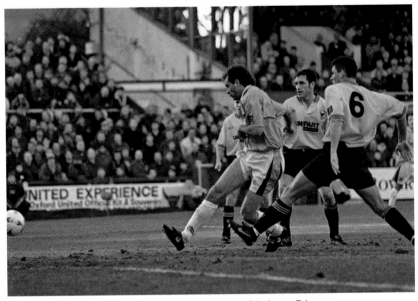

**Back in the groove:** On target at Oxford United during a 4-1 victory, February 1997; (below left) the winner against Oldham Athletic a month later, and (below right) celebrating my penalty against Middlesbrough, December 1997

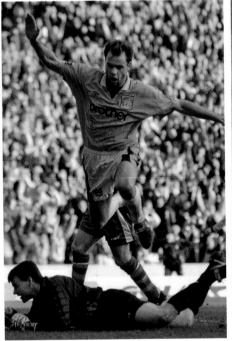

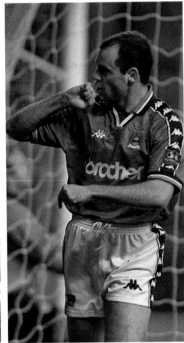

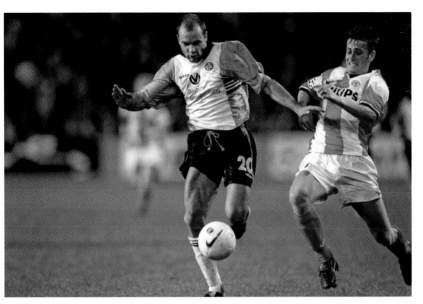

**Champions League performer:** (Above and below left) On the attack for Kaiserslautern during the 2-1 victory over PSV Eindhoven in October 1998, and (below right) celebrating one of my three goals against HJK Helsinki, December 1998

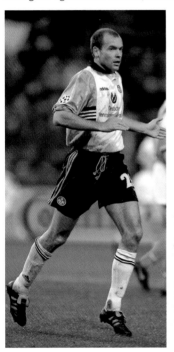

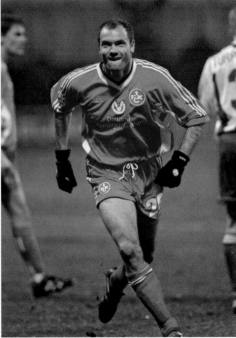

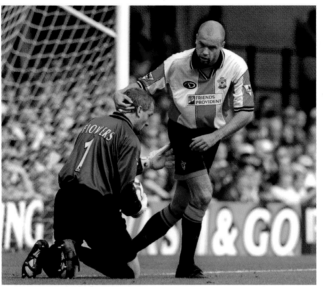

**Uwe Saint:** A friendly greeting for Leicester City goalkeeper Tim Flowers, September 2000

**Baggies blow:** An unwelcome mark from my brief spell at West Bromwich Albion, in a fiery 1-0 victory at Birmingham City in November 2001

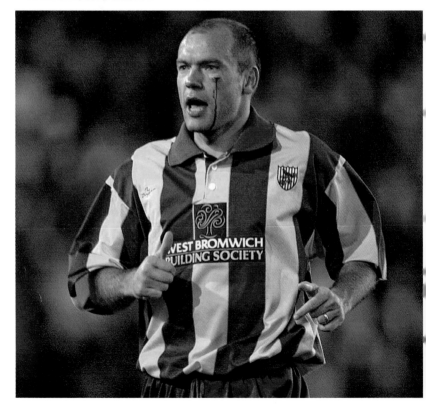

The injury aside, it had been an incredible first full season for me in England. I loved the city, my team-mates were perfect, the supporters were incredible and in Brian Horton, I had a manager who believed and trusted in me. What more could I have asked for?

But things were about to change. Five games from the end of the campaign we knew that a strong end to the season could see us still finish in the top 10. We were away to Blackburn Rovers, live on Sky Sports, and a win for Rovers would virtually guarantee them the title and leave them possibly nine points clear of Manchester United with four games to go. We'd won just three of our 18 away games while they'd taken 46 from a possible 54 at Ewood Park – it looked a home banker on paper.

However, we were really up for it that night and beat them 3-2 to move within two points of 10th-placed Arsenal. We played the kind of football we knew we were capable of under Horton and I felt it was a huge statement that we could outplay and beat the champions-elect in their own backyard. With one or two tweaks, I felt we weren't far off being a top-six side. We were on a high after the game – even if we had done United a massive favour – and we headed home really looking forward to a strong finish and the prospect of an exciting 1995/96 season.

When the team coach headed for a pub in Haydock on the way home, like everyone else, I thought the gaffer was taking us for a few pints to celebrate a good night's work, but we were taken into a side room and the doors were closed. The room fell silent and the gaffer told us he would be leaving the club at the end of the season. Here was the man who had brought me to England, given me my opportunity and helped me flourish, and now he was leaving? I was devastated. We had been a bit up and down that season but we could still finish in mid-table, which would have meant progress after the previous year's relegation battle, so I couldn't understand why he was leaving.

There was nothing any of us could do because the chairman wanted a change and had told him he would be bringing in someone else. Change is part and parcel of football and we would have to get on with it, but we were all gutted. We drew our next two games and lost the final two to end a disappointing 17th, and I put that down to the flat atmosphere at the club.

The traditional end-of-season dinner was very sombre and something I think we'd have happily avoided on this occasion, but it turned out to be a very proud evening for me as it was revealed I was the City fans' Player of the Year for 1994/95. I felt honoured, and the bond between me and the supporters amazed me. They sang my name three or four times in every game, they'd adopted me as one of their own, believed in me and were behind me 100 per cent. With their backing, I felt I was playing the best football of my career. I'd left my comfort zone, my friends and family and everything I knew behind, yet I was thriving in England. The award meant so much as it was my first full season at the club and it meant even more because I'd been up against Paul Walsh, Niall Quinn and Peter Beagrie, all of whom would have been worthy winners.

So while that gave me a much-needed boost, the departure of Gaudino was another disappointment on the back of Horton's departure. I knew Francis Lee had been trying to sign him throughout his loan spell, but for one reason or another, he never managed to make it happen. Maurizio decided to move to Club America in Mexico, enticed by a great contract and a different way of life. Years later, I met him again and he still regretted leaving City. It was, he told me, the biggest mistake of his life. He'd put the thought of sunshine, lifestyle and money ahead of his career and he's regretted it ever since.

So we needed a new manager and no doubt that meant there would have to be changes behind the scenes and probably on the playing side, too. I wondered who would come in next as I boarded the plane home to Germany for the summer and where – and if – I would fit in his plans.

# 10

# Ganz neues Ballspiel

## (Whole new Ball game)

The first time I saw a T-shirt with 'Uwe's grandad bombed Old Trafford' I had to smile. I was learning English and both understood and enjoyed English humour, so I totally got it. The German media were quick to pick up on it and I was being told that I couldn't allow that to happen and that they were making fun of our country's history. I was interviewed for one paper and they said I must be upset and depressed about what was happening and I told them I was anything but. Totally the opposite in fact. I told them it was just English humour, that's the way it was and it was nothing more than harmless fun. There were 5,000 T-shirts printed and they sold the lot, so it was a good idea by somebody! Besides, if I hadn't been accepted as one of their own, I don't think there's any way those T-shirts would have appeared.

By this time, I'd also been given the nickname 'Der Bomber' in the Manchester Evening News, which was very flattering. Gerd Muller was the original Der Bomber, but I couldn't compare myself with him – nowhere near, to be honest – but I liked it. Who wouldn't?

I had a great summer with Cecilie and was looking forward to returning for pre-season training. Shortly before we were due to return, City announced Alan Ball would be the next manager. I knew he was a famous name in England and that he'd done quite well with Southampton the season before, but other than that, I didn't know that much about his management skills.

I think it's fair to say he probably wasn't the person City supporters were hoping would take over, but he was a World Cup winner and you couldn't argue with someone who had played almost 1,000 career games and won 72 caps for his country. He was close friends with Francis Lee as well and I know there was some urgency because we'd been without a manager for six or seven weeks. Of course, we were eager to find out what he was like, which style of play he wanted us to adopt and what sort of players, if any, he was going to bring in.

Ball had sold Paul Walsh when he was Portsmouth manager, so there were rumours very early on that Walshy was going to be sold. At the time I thought this couldn't possibly be true. We'd struck up a really productive partnership and he was hugely popular with the fans and in the dressing room. He'd just had one of the best seasons of his career, so I hoped it was a rumour and no more.

We all met Ball for the first time when we returned for pre-season training at the university grounds City used as a kind of base camp. We were looking forward to seeing what he had to say and were curious about how he saw things developing, and which system we would play. He gathered us all together and during his first talk he mentioned his World Cup winner's medal, which I had no problem with. It didn't affect me because I respected his achievements and was open to new ideas, but it didn't go down too well with all the lads, particularly the more experienced players in the squad who wondered why he'd mentioned something everyone was already aware of.

Things started badly for me and maybe I should have taken it as a sign of things to come when I picked up an injury in early pre-season. It couldn't have come at a worse time. It was looking like I'd be out for a month at a point when I had to make sure I was at the forefront of the manager's thoughts. In my mind, the only way I could speed up the process of healing was to fly back to Germany and visit Dr. Hans-Wilhelm Müller-Wohlfahrt, who was based in Munich. He was the club doctor at Bayern, a world leader in the treatment of sports injuries, although some of his methods are considered somewhat controversial. Francis Lee very kindly paid for me to go home and at the time, it was quite unusual for a player to leave the country to seek treatment, but I had such confidence in Dr. Müller-Wohlfahrt and his team that I honestly thought there was a chance I'd be fit for the start of the season under his care.

As he was unavailable, I went to see Dr. Friedrich, who was a protégé of Muller-Wohlfahrt. The reputation of the clinic was renowned throughout Germany so I knew I was in good hands and, sure enough, within a fortnight, I was well ahead of schedule and on course for the opening match of the season.

While I was away, Georgi Kinkladze joined the club. All we knew of Georgi was that he'd played for Georgia against Wales and given Vinnie Jones a terrible time and scored a fantastic goal. He had been to Saarbrucken in Germany but things hadn't worked out for him there, and so he'd gone back to Georgia. I'd heard he was a very skilful player and was looking forward to playing alongside him.

The first training session I saw him play in convinced me he was the real deal. At 21, he was stocky – maybe even a little overweight – but he had great vision, technique and balance, so he was an exciting addition to the team. What I couldn't envisage was where he would fit in because his ability was quite unique. I could see Georgi was going to give the manager one or two problems – not in a negative way, just where he would get the best out of him, because he could have played on the wing, through the middle or as a second striker.

I returned from Germany ready for action but with no pre-season under my belt and no match fitness to speak of. I won my place in the starting line-up for the home game with Tottenham and scored our goal – a header from a hopeful Ian Brightwell cross – in a 1-1 draw. I'd achieved my aim, but at what cost? I was nowhere near ready for the demands of a Premiership season and it would soon show as the team began to struggle. I scored again in a 2-1 defeat at Coventry City and then the goals dried up, not only for me, but for the whole team.

We had no recognisable formation to speak of and there was general confusion in our play. Unbelievably, Walshy was sold to Portsmouth and in return we got Gerry Creaney who, with respect, was nowhere near the player Paul was. I thought it was a poor piece of business by the club and those thoughts were echoed by our fans, who were also mystified. In many ways it put a huge question mark over Ball's judgement in the minds of our fans and some of the players. I had tried to talk Walshy out of it, but he told me the writing had been on the wall since Ball arrived because I think there was some history between them. He didn't want to go and even at 33, he was in great shape and the irony was, if any player would benefit from having a talent like Kinkladze behind him, it was Paul Walsh. But it was too late and he headed back to Pompey where we'd signed him from just 18 months before. Our loss was very much their gain.

Again, I was devastated to lose a close friend on the back of Brian Horton's departure. Just a couple of games into the season there was already real unrest in the dressing room. There was no direction or real style of play that we were being asked to play and it showed quickly on the pitch, where we were all over the place at times. In November, Martin 'Buster' Phillips signed for £500,000 from Exeter City. He was just a kid and I was astonished when Ball said at his press conference that Phillips would be Britain's first £10m player. What a statement to make, and the pressure and expectation it instantly put on his young shoulders didn't help him at all. How could he ever live up to that billing?

He was a nice lad with a lot of talent and a fantastic family around him, but he would never be able to cope with that sort of expectation at a club the size of City. Every time he played, he tried too hard because he was attempting to justify the manager's words, but with a big, expectant crowd watching his every move, he was doomed to fail. He needed to be nurtured and gradually eased into the first-team but it was too late to change what had already been said.

We continued our poor form in the league and even in the League Cup, we drew the first leg of our tie with League Two side Wycombe 0-0. There was a massive argument among the players after the match as the unrest that had been boiling under the surface finally exploded. It wasn't a happy camp but it was borne out of frustration more than anything else.

I broke my own personal drought with a couple of goals in the return match at Maine Road, a 4-0 win, and it at least brought some relief. It was only a brief respite, however, as we sank to the foot of the table and things got much worse before they got better. We went to Liverpool in the next round of the cup and we were soundly beaten 4-0, but in the league game, also at Anfield three day later, we were thrashed 6-0.

Our fans had been amazing at Anfield and were still singing when Liverpool scored their sixth of the afternoon, so at the end of the match, having been totally outplayed from start to finish, I went over to them and threw my boots into the crowd as a gift to express my personal thanks for sticking with us when it would have been easy to go the other way. I couldn't believe they'd been so supportive so I wanted to give them something back. I felt the boots were jinxed anyway as I'd never scored in them, but the media turned it around and suggested there was something other than goodwill in my gesture. One headline read 'Uwe gives City fans the boot' and suggested I'd had enough of the City fans, which was ridiculous. I made my feelings clear in the local media but it was a reminder of how even the simplest gesture could be turned on its head when things were going badly.

So our Premiership record at this point was: Played: 11, Won: 0, Drawn: 2, Lost: 9, Goals scored: 3, Conceded: 21.

We were dead men walking and were already being written off in the press as relegation certainties. I wondered if the manager hadn't been such good friends with the chairman, would he have survived the sack?

It wasn't all Ball's fault. I wasn't playing as well as I could because of my interrupted pre-season, but I still had confidence and belief and I gave it everything each time I went out.

In my opinion, we were changing the formation too often and nobody knew their role or had time to bed into a position. On one occasion I was put on the right-wing, Niall Quinn on the left and Georgi Kinkladze went down the middle but whatever we tried just wasn't working. Now Quinny's no winger and neither am I, so that didn't last long! Sometimes we had no wingers at all and played everything down the middle and I felt there was too much focus on trying to find the right position for Georgi – who was our most talented player – rather than what was best for the team.

Ball was attempting to find a way to integrate Georgi, which was the right thing to do, but he appeared to lose sight of the bigger picture. Instead of maybe holding his hands up and saying that he'd made some mistakes in those first few months, the manager started blaming me and Niall Quinn for the lack of goals. I was angry that he was criticising us in public but I must add that none of this had anything to do with Georgi who was as good as gold, a fantastic talent and a really nice guy.

There were some big characters in our dressing room, including Tony Coton, Quinny, Keith Curle, Peter Beagrie and Terry Phelan and it's fair to say they didn't see eye-to-eye with Ball.

Perhaps they feared their time at the club was nearing an end? I was happy to hold my hands up and admit I wasn't where I wanted to be. I simply wasn't firing on all cylinders. Without Walsh and the injured Beags, we'd lost two thirds of an attack that had been so effective the previous season and there was now a lack of understanding in how we played as a team, with the new players not fully integrated.

But I still believed we had too much quality to be cut adrift at the foot of the Premiership so the problem for me was the lack of direction and some confusion in our play. The training was a little one-dimensional, too, but then, seemingly against the odds, we started to win games and during November, we won four games and drew one – a complete turnaround in fortunes. Alan Ball even won the Manager of the Month award. All our wins had been 1-0 so scoring goals was still our Achilles heel, and I was still looking for my first goal in 13 Premiership games. I managed just two in our first 15 matches and the drought was right up there with the worst runs of my career at Nürnberg, but the fans still gave me that belief in my own abilities, sang my name and were with me, so I still thought I would score each time I went out.

The football wasn't flowing, but we'd dug in and there was finally some light at the end of the tunnel, but still many questions needed to be answered. The purple patch turned out to be no more than an anomaly as we took just one point out of our next 12. I was happy to score in the 1-1 draw with Nottingham Forest, but aside from a 2-1 win over West Ham, it was a miserable Christmas and New Year period.

The FA Cup at least provided a welcome distraction and we saw off Leicester City after a replay and then Coventry City, again after a replay. We were into the last 16 but pulled out an away tie at Manchester United in the fifth round. While it meant it would be a fantastic occasion for our fans, it was the last match we needed at that point.

We would be taking 12,000 fans to Old Trafford and we thought we could go there and give a decent account of ourselves, maybe even bring them back to our place. Okay, we hadn't won there for 22 years, but at the end of the day it was just 11 versus 11 and we had a chance.

I'd started to understand Georgi a lot better and he'd really found his role in the team. We also knew a lot more about what he was about and it would show in this game. Nobody gave us a chance at Old Trafford but once we walked out at the Stretford End and saw our fans banked away at the other end, we puffed out our chests and, if nothing else, we'd make sure we gave United a game for them. It was the most amazing atmosphere I'd experienced with our fans incredible from start to finish. I knew it would be a career high if I could score in front of them, so when I was given the chance, I knew I had to take it.

Georgi got the ball just over the halfway line, span his marker and spotted my run. He played the ball through to leave me clear on goal. Peter Schmeichel raced off his line to the edge of the box so it was now or never. He was almost up to me and in a split second, I knew I either had to go around him or try to chip him. I had to go with my instinct and I knew he didn't really think I'd try and chip him so I deftly scooped the ball over his head. As it went over his outstretched arms, it brushed his fingertips on its way towards the goal where it bounced once before entering the empty net.

The City fans erupted, going crazy behind the goal and I ran towards them and celebrated before I was mobbed. It is still one of my favourite career moments. Sadly, United were awarded a soft penalty before the break – the sort you only get at home with a big crowd behind you – from which they scored. They then added another in the second half to go through 2-1.

I was gutted because we'd been worth a replay and perhaps more. It was hard to take solace from the fact we'd shown a lot of character and had pushed them all the way. The bottom line was we'd lost to United and were out of the cup. Now all we had ahead of us was a relegation battle, but if we could show the same fight as we had done at Old Trafford, then we'd give ourselves a real chance.

# 11

# Kein Weg zurück?

## (No way back?)

I'd crept into double figures by the time the Maine Road Manchester derby came around. Since the turn of the year we'd won three, drawn six and lost four of our 13 matches, and also started scoring and conceding more goals. We were unbeaten at home in nine games in all competitions, and a 2-1 win over fellow strugglers Southampton had given us renewed hope of beating the drop.

I think everyone who was at Maine Road that day against Southampton had witnessed something very special with the unforgettable goal Kinky scored, him beating maybe five players before deftly chipping the ball over Dave Beasant. At the time I didn't realise quite how good the goal was, but watching it on video the next day, I was amazed at how technically brilliant it was. For me, it was as good as Diego Maradona's solo effort against England in 1986 – perhaps even better – and it underlined what a talent Georgi was. At his best, he was untouchable and at times it was almost like watching a ballet dancer. It was a pleasure to play alongside him when he was in full flow.

However, instead of building on that win, we followed it with a 4-2 defeat at West Ham and a 1-1 draw with Bolton. I hadn't played particularly well in the Bolton game but was happy with my overall form and contribution to the team.

Mikhail Kavelashvili had arrived just before the transfer window shut in the week building up to the derby to give Alan Ball more attacking options, which was fine by me as I welcomed competition for places. Mikhail was a Georgia international and a good friend of Georgi's, and the Manchester Evening News had suggested that Kavelashvili would perhaps start up front against United instead of me. I doubted that would happen because to throw a player into a game of that magnitude was a massive risk, but I wasn't certain if it was just speculation and paper talk. I'd had my disagreements with the manager but nothing out of the ordinary, so I felt comfortable enough to ask him if there was any truth in the rumours at the Wednesday Platt Lane training session.

I hadn't been dropped since I joined City and if it was about to happen for a game of that stature, I wanted to get my head around it, so I asked Ball straight out if it was true. The derby was the highlight of the season and I didn't want to be angry and disappointed before the match because I'd be too pumped up and not in a good place. If I had a day or two to deal with it, I could then focus on being on the bench and being ready, if and when needed. It was nothing to do with an inflated ego, just my own way of dealing with things so I could ultimately give my best for the team.

As it was, I had nothing to worry about. Ball gave me 100 per cent assurance that I would be playing and a 100 per cent assurance that I was still his main striker, so I left the office feeling good and looking forward to the match. I actually thought it was a good piece of man-management because he'd built me up and given me the reassurances I wanted to hear ahead of what was a huge game for us.

It's fair to say that the manager and I were never close. He'd blamed me publicly for the lack of goals, saying I wasn't scoring as many as I had the previous season and indicating that was why we were struggling. While it was true I had scored half as many as I had the previous campaign, the whole team had scored half as many, too, so it had been unfair and certainly hadn't motivated me or Niall Quinn and a few others who'd been criticised in the media. Yes, I wanted to prove him wrong, but he just had a knack of saying the wrong thing at the wrong time. But I was professional and never let the criticism affect me on the pitch. We still communicated, hence our pre-derby chat, and I had no personal axe to grind with him, but what happened next completely moved the goalposts for me and, regrettably, it did become personal – very personal.

I left home for Maine Road and was in a very positive frame of mind. I was desperate to get among the United defence, ruffle a few feathers and to help us carry on where we'd left off in the FA Cup tie at Old Trafford, where we still felt a deep sense of injustice. I parked up, signed a few autographs outside the main entrance and headed for the dressing room. I opened the door and straight away saw my shirt was hanging up ready – where Kavelashvili's was. That's how I discovered I wasn't in the starting line-up.

It was the first time since I'd joined City that I had been dropped, and I was absolutely furious because I'd tried to avoid this situation by asking the manager whether I would be starting or not. Had he told me I would be sub, I would have been angry and disappointed, but I would have dealt with it and had time to get over it and re-focus.

I couldn't hide my anger or disappointment and I felt badly let down by Ball. I was well aware how I would react to this kind of situation which is why I'd taken steps to diffuse it, yet here I was, unable to conceal my feelings. I was just so emotionally charged on matchdays – and always had been – and I needed some sort of outlet, to unleash all my anger and energy. The manager didn't speak to me or explain why he'd changed his mind and I left the dressing room to try and cool down.

I got changed and took my place on the subs' bench before kick-off and tried to calm myself down. Eric Cantona put United ahead early on from the penalty spot, but on 39 minutes, Kavelashvili equalised with a great goal. It was then that I thought, hmmm… maybe my time at City might be coming to an end? I'd seen Paul Walsh and Garry Flitcroft go – among others – and now I thought that the manager wanted me out.

I couldn't argue with the way Mikhail had started his City career. But had the manager intended to play me as a sub all along to bring things to a head? I'll never know the answer to that because Alan is no longer with us to speak for himself. I can only give my side of events.

Andy Cole scored within a minute of our equaliser and after

around 70 minutes, I was told I was coming on. I was desperate to prove the manager wrong and though he gave me some instructions as I waited to go on, I didn't hear a thing. I was too far gone and lost in my own world. I was full of anger but at the same time completely motivated, so when I picked up the ball just past our halfway line, nothing was going to stop me. I powered forward, checked inside and hit the ball from 20 yards with such venom and energy that Schmeichel didn't have a chance. It was a shot filled with rage but I hit it so cleanly it was a goal as soon as it left my boot.

I set off to celebrate in front of the North Stand but my reaction from then on is something I still deeply regret to this day. I headed towards Ball in the dug-out and I think Nigel Clough, who sprinted towards me, could see what my intentions were but I shrugged him off as he attempted to hold me back. I pointed the name on my shirt in front of our bench, lost in the moment and I just wish I could wind back the clock and erase that moment from time.

It was unprofessional and there was no justification for it. My only defence is had the manager told me sooner, I would have been over it by the time I scored. I've always worn my heart on my sleeve, it's just the way I'm made and I didn't believe the world revolved around Uwe Rosler – far from it – but I should have known better.

Ryan Giggs scored six minutes later and we ended up losing 3-2 but, for me, the damage was done. I made things even worse with a stupid interview I gave Match of the Day after the match. I was still raging and should never have spoken to anyone. Today, the club's press officer would never have let me talk to the media in such an emotional state, but back then, it was different.

# KNOCKING DOWN WALLS

When I was asked if there was a problem between me and Alan Ball, I said. "Yes, there is a massive problem between me and the manager. I'm not playing for him. I'm playing for this football club, my team-mates and our supporters, but not for Alan Ball." I felt my time was over so I just said it the way I felt it was. I went into the dressing room, had a shower and didn't speak to anyone before storming out and heading home.

As I gradually calmed down, I realised what I'd done and called my agent to tell him. Then I saw myself on Match of the Day and saw the interview and felt even more embarrassed. I'd been stupid and could have no real complaints if I'd been shown the door. If I have one regret from that whole sorry episode it is that, in later years, I never had the chance to apologise to Alan for that incident, and that is something I regret.

On Monday morning I arrived for training and waited for the call to see the manager and presumably begin a disciplinary hearing of some kind, but he didn't mention anything. We trained as normal and nothing happened afterwards, either. I wasn't fined and it was something that was never discussed again, which I found mystifying. Whether Ball had decided he'd been in the wrong and was willing to let it go, or simply didn't think it merited any action, I don't know. There was no sit-down, no confrontation and no two weeks' wages fine – nothing. I hadn't been put on the transfer list and Francis Lee, who I had a very good relationship with – his son, Gary, was and still is my best friend in England – hadn't called me in either. I'd been prepared to take my medicine and face the consequences of such a public show of defiance, but it was all brushed under the carpet and forgotten.

So we moved on. I was restored to the starting line-up and it was as though nothing had ever happened – unless the plan had been to avoid further upset and deal with it at the end of the season. Either way, I had no idea.

We now had four games to save ourselves and a 3-0 defeat at Wimbledon didn't help matters, but we won our next two games with a goal from me and Steve Lomas enough to beat Sheffield Wednesday and Aston Villa respectively. We'd pretty much gone from as good as being down after Wimbledon to having a real chance of staying up on the final day. All we needed to do was better either Coventry City or Southampton's result and we'd stay up.

We all went into the final match on 37 points, but our goal difference was seven worse off. Coventry were at home to Leeds United and Southampton were at home to Wimbledon – both very winnable games against lower mid-table sides, whereas we hosted Liverpool, who couldn't finish any higher or lower than third place. A win wouldn't guarantee our survival, but it would give us the best chance of staying up and Liverpool, in theory, had nothing to play for other than pride.

The build-up to the game was huge, with various permutations and scenarios mulled over in the press. But we still felt confident that we could pull off what would be, considering the awful start we'd made to the season, the great escape.

The game began and we were extremely edgy, making stupid mistakes and unforced errors. I had two good chances – one hit the post and the other went wide – and by half-time, we found ourselves 2-0 down after Steve Lomas put through his own goal and Ian Rush tapped home another. At the break the manager blamed me for us being behind, but I'd heard it all before so I walked out of the dressing room to refocus. I felt I was certain to be substituted after what the manager had said, so when the lads came down the tunnel I asked Kit Symons if I was still involved and he said I was. I was surprised, but at least I still had a chance at helping influence our future.

The other teams were both drawing 0-0, so it wasn't over yet, and on 71 minutes, Georgi Kinkladze was brought down in the box and the ref awarded a penalty. Nobody was going to take the ball away from me and though the pressure was intense, I hammered the ball home to make it 1-2. Eight minutes later, Symons arrived in the box from nowhere to make it 2-2 and with 11 minutes remaining, we were back in with a real chance of surviving.

The atmosphere was electric as we poured forward looking for a third. Niall Quinn had taken a knock and had been subbed so was watching the game from the physio room. He knew the situation was that Coventry and Southampton were still drawing 0-0 and we needed a third goal, but with a few minutes remaining, we got an instruction from the bench to hold the ball in the corner and waste time as Coventry were now losing, which was obviously not true – not that we knew. Lomas and myself both headed towards the corner of the pitch over the next few moments trying to run the clock down – and that's when Quinny raced from the physio room and up the touchline dressed only in a towel and yelled at us that we needed another goal, but we'd already wasted a few valuable moments.

A minute later and the referee blew for full-time before we could really do anything about it. That whole charade summed up our season and while we may well have not scored another goal even if we'd been given the correct information, we'd have given it a good go and who knows what might have happened?

Instead, we'd been relegated and while the table doesn't lie, we should have been well away from the bottom three with the squad we had.

We'd had more than enough quality within the squad, yet between the players and the manager we hadn't been able to save ourselves, so the blame needed to be shared equally. We were completely gutted and left the pitch. We got changed and went home emotionally and physically drained, unable to absorb what had just happened. Everyone was devastated and it was without doubt the worst moment of my playing career. There was no finger-pointing, nothing.

We all wanted to get away as quickly as possible, and after the MCFC Player of the Year awards the following day, I did just that. I'd scored 13 goals in total and still managed to end the season as top scorer for the second year running. While I hadn't had a fantastic season, I still felt I'd played my last game for City because of what had gone on in the previous 12 months. I knew playing under Alan Ball again would be difficult after everything that had happened, so while leaving was the last thing I wanted to do, I accepted there may be no other option.

# 12

## Das Herz regiert meinen Kopf

### (Heart ruling my head)

I still harboured hopes of making the 1996 European Championships, particularly as it was being held in England, but I knew that the prospect of playing in the second tier was going to make that virtually impossible. How could I compete with scoring goals against – with the greatest respect – Southend United and Oxford United when the guys I was up against for a place in the German squad were scoring in the Bundesliga and the Champions League on a regular basis? It didn't take a genius to work out that unless I moved on there was no chance for me playing at major championships or making an impression of any sort on the international stage.

Considering we'd been relegated, I received something of surprise a call in the summer from Germany boss Berti Vogts who
told me, in his opinion, I had to leave City if I was to have any
chance with the national team by either playing for a Premiership club or return to the Bundesliga. I knew he'd had scouts
watching me over the past 12 months and I had an important
decision to make.

I felt sure the club would look to sell me so I spoke to my agent
and had a chat about how things were going. The club had
made a statement that they would be sticking with Ball for the
new season but I also knew that if I said I wanted to leave, it
would look like I was a rat deserting a sinking ship and that was
the last thing I wanted. I loved being a City player and I doubted I would ever find the kind of relationship I had with the
supporters anywhere else – no amount of money could replace
that. I needed some time to think and for the intense feeling of
disappointment to dissipate before I did anything, so I went on
holiday with Cecilie, then spent some time in Germany before
returning for pre-season training.

Quinny, a great friend and team-mate, had gone to Sunderland. I think he'd had enough and was ready for a new challenge and, frankly, he was too good for Division One. Peter
Beagrie, another guy I thought the world of and who'd become
a close friend, had gone to Bradford City and Keith Curle had
joined Wolves, too, so we'd lost some great dressing room leaders as well as three very good players. I think everyone expected
Kinkladze to move on, too, with Celtic, Liverpool and Barce-
lona all rumoured to be interested, but I think Francis Lee convinced him to give it one more season.

The players we were bringing in were not the same quality

as the ones we were losing, and there were a number of lower league lads brought in. Martin Phillips, tipped by Ball to be the first £10m player, was now almost a permanent fixture in the reserves and a number of loan players arrived to add to a squad that already had almost 40 senior pros in it.

We were expected to blow the league away but we were mentally nowhere near ready for the challenge ahead, and we'd lost too much experience too quickly. We needed people who knew how to get out of that league and the truth was, we had nobody who fitted that description on our books. I felt there were too many players from overseas who weren't up to the demands of second-tier football, because it's a completely different challenge to the Premiership.

For pre-season we went to Ireland and China, but it was something of a disaster from start to finish. There was a lot of negativity in the camp and too much water had gone under the bridge. Talking of water, we flew to China to play three games but we'd been there just a couple of days when we were told the tour would have to be abandoned due to the extensive flooding around the country.

In Ireland, things happened that shouldn't have happened at a top professional football club preparing for such an important season. Discipline and the standards of professionalism were at an all-time low and, for me, it was no surprise that things quickly deteriorated on the pitch. Even though we started with a 1-0 win over Ipswich Town, we were unconvincing. If Ball was to continue as manager, we needed a flawless start and a midweek defeat at Bolton suggested it was going to be a much tougher season than everyone had envisaged.

One good signing we did make was Paul Dickov, who arrived

in time to play in our next game away to Stoke City. He reminded me a lot of Paul Walsh with his style of play, energy and
tireless work-rate. He was aggressive but a good footballer and
someone I knew I'd enjoy playing alongside. He was aware that
we'd need to fight and scrap rather than play our way out of the
division straight from the off. In future years we'd become close
friends and we got along well from the very beginning.

We went to the Victoria Ground and ran out to see 5,000 City
fans behind one of the goals, which told you everything you
needed to know about them. I scored that day, but we found
ourselves 2-1 down in the second half and you could sense
something in the air. I believe both sets of fans were calling for
Alan Ball to be sacked – the Stoke fans hadn't enjoyed his stint
there as manager and the City fans had endured enough. We
couldn't find a way back into the game and after the final whis-
tle you could sense something was going to happen. There was
a certain amount of inevitability about the fate of the manager
and by the start of the following week, Ball was sacked. Despite
our past differences, it gave me no pleasure to see him relieved
of his duties – that may sound a little odd, but it is how I felt.

I was interested to see who would come in and Crystal Palace
manager Dave Bassett turned down the chance to take over, if
I recall correctly, because he felt the club was in disarray on and
off the pitch. The biggest losers were our fans and the football
club because we were out of the top flight for the first time in
seven years and seemingly heading nowhere.

We had six weeks or so under caretaker-manager Asa Hart-
ford while the club sought a suitable replacement. Asa was now
part of the coaching staff, having rejoined the club where he'd
spent two successful stints as a player. I really liked Asa, he wore

his heart on his sleeve – something I could relate to – and we had much in common. I hoped he would be given the opportunity to maybe take the job until the end of the season. However, our results were very inconsistent and certainly not those of a team with serious promotion ambitions. By the start of October, we'd dropped to 14th in the table and were nine points behind leaders Norwich City, so while things weren't going well, with a new man and new impetus, we still had enough quality to make a challenge for promotion.

I was scoring goals and we were slowly adjusting to being the big fish in a small pond. Everyone wanted to beat Manchester City. We played Lincoln City in the League Cup and lost 4-1 at Sincil Bank and then 1-0 in the return at Maine Road. We needed some direction and guidance – and quickly. We were still playing in front of crowds of nearly 30,000 at Maine Road, and some of the lads we'd brought in were finding it difficult to cope with the pressure and expectations that came with being at a club of City's size. Our fans quite rightly expected more and deserved better.

Finally, Steve Coppell was appointed after leaving his position as director of football at Crystal Palace and from day one, the training improved markedly. The sessions were very good, enjoyable and varied. We practised a lot on attacking and on finishing which, for me, was perfect, and I felt he was the right man to take us forward.

Steve was quiet and humble but I think he quickly realised the magnitude of the situation he'd found himself in and after just 33 days, he resigned, unwilling to let the pressure and expectation take its toll on his health. We were all stunned and also back to square one. Our results under Coppell had been patchy but I felt we'd been heading in the right direction. His assistant, Phil Neal, took over and we now had our fourth manager of the season – and it was only November!

Our form under Neal was abysmal and we lost seven out of our next 10 games, effectively ending any hopes we'd had of going up that season. We were now just fourth from bottom and looking more likely to go down again, which seemed unthinkable. It was chaotic and things only started to settle when Frank Clark took over just after Christmas. I liked Clark immediately and he was the calming influence we desperately needed. He was very experienced and he spoke a lot to me, gave me advice and I learned a lot from him.

I began scoring freely again with eight goals during a six-week spell after Christmas. Clark wanted me to sign a new contract and I felt settled and happy again with the whole team responding and going on an unbeaten run of nine games in the league. I was enjoying every training session and Kevin Horlock joined us, who proved a good, talented player who knew what was needed to get out of the division.

I'd also struck up a real understanding with Paul Dickov and especially Georgi. I knew that if I made certain runs, he'd find me. A lot of people remember him making a goal for me against Southend, when I ran up to him and took a bow in front of the North Stand. It was an appreciation of his vision and skill and what had been a forgettable campaign was ending on a real high. By mid-April, we'd lost just two of the 16 league games under Clark and had we had him in charge a month or so earlier, I honestly think we'd have had a good chance of making the play-offs. As it was, we were probably six points adrift of being able to make a serious late challenge.

# KNOCKING DOWN WALLS

Before the end of the season, Clark informed me that he wanted to commit my future to City and sign a new contract, and that things would be discussed during the summer. I would have been more than happy to sign there and then. I'd missed my chance of forcing my way into the German European Championships squad, which was no great surprise as the moment I decided I would stay at City, I knew my chances were as good as over with the national team. I had enjoyed myself so much again though. I had finished as top scorer for the third season in a row with 17 goals from 49 games, and felt the instability would surely come to an end at the club and we'd be in good stead for a promotion push the following season.

Clark then asked me to travel to our last away game of the season at Norwich, despite the fact I'd picked up an injury. At the team hotel on the Friday evening before the game we spoke together, along with my agent Jerome Anderson, and agreed verbally on a new four-year contract which would be finalised on our return after the summer break. I couldn't have been happier. City were my club, the fans were always behind me and I was also due to marry Cecilie, who was pregnant with our first child. We were moving into our first house at long last and in my mind, I wanted to end my career with City.

So while I was settled and focused for the new season, it came as a surprise when I heard Lee Bradbury had been signed for more than £3m from Portsmouth. At that time, it was a massive amount of money, especially for a club outside the top flight, but I knew I had a new deal to come so I wasn't unduly concerned. I had no idea of the drama that actually lay ahead...

# 13

# Der Anfang vom Ende

## (The beginning of the end)

We returned for pre-season and headed off for an unremarkable tour of Scotland. Franny Lee had again convinced Georgi to stay for one more season so we were well placed to have a good go at winning promotion. I waited for a call from the boss to finalise the new deal, but for one reason or another it didn't happen, instead becoming quickly overshadowed by the appalling start we made to the season. It was inexplicable. We won just three of our opening 17 games, and had slipped into the bottom three of the table.

City had also received an offer for me from Everton, managed by Joe Royle, but I think their valuation differed from City's and nothing seemed to progress. It probably didn't help that I picked up an injury in September, and soon after my first son was born at Stepping Hill Hospital so my focus was elsewhere.

Besides, I was too thrilled to be a dad for the first time and was just happy my son was healthy and finally here. I insisted we call him Tony after Tony Book, who I had so much respect for at City. It wouldn't be the first child we named after a City legend, either! I had plenty on my mind and the contract situation seemed to become less important for a while, though with a young son to now take care of, it would certainly take precedence in the months to come.

Bradbury was also ruled out for several months so our first choice forward line was effectively ruled out. I'd missed the 3-1 win over Nottingham Forest due to the birth of Tony, and I was put on the bench for a few games afterwards before a behind-closed-doors friendly was arranged against a team of Italian players hoping to win a contract in England. During the game, one of their players went over the top as he challenged me and badly damaged my ankle ligaments. It was a career-changing tackle because I was ruled out for three months, which effectively ended Everton's interest in me and I returned to Germany for treatment. Meanwhile, all hell broke loose back at Maine Road.

Francis Lee left as chairman after fan protests escalated and John Wardle stepped up in his place. We were back in total disarray again and by the time I returned in early December, we were again looking at a relegation battle. It was just a matter of time before Frank Clark resigned and shortly after Christmas, he did exactly that. I still hadn't signed a new deal but when Joe Royle was announced as the new manager, I felt confident that we had brought in someone who had belief in my ability. I thought things would be sorted out quickly.

Joe told me he was looking forward to working with me but that I'd still have to prove myself to him, just as everyone else would have to before any contracts were agreed. I had been top scorer for the past three seasons but I understood everyone was starting with a blank sheet of paper and that Joe wouldn't be solely concentrating on me. He had a lot of sorting out to do, with a lot of highly paid pros on the books – enough for three teams in fact, and we had a squad of 50, which was ridiculous.

I felt there were other things going on in the background to do with finances and, again, began to wonder what the future held. Royle tried to steady the ship and brought in more players who knew the lower leagues such as Shaun Goater, Richard Jobson, Jamie Pollock and also Peter Beardsley, who may have been nearing the end of his career but who was still a class act.

Joe also took what he believed to be decisive action by dropping Kinkladze in mid-February – a brave call to make on a player so popular with our supporters. I think he felt that numerous managers had tried to figure out how best to utilise Georgi's undoubted talents with various systems and formations, and he just felt none of them had worked. Maybe Georgi and I had both outstayed our welcome because we'd both slipped down the divisions as regular staples in the team. While we'd done our best and given everything, the truth was that the team was facing relegation to the third tier of English football for the first time.

We were losing against teams like Stockport County and Port Vale and being outfought by clubs who knew how to scrap and fight for points, as well as saving their best for when we rolled into town. Our aura may not have been what it once was, but we were still a prize scalp to some clubs who knew they probably wouldn't get many chances to play us at home and away. We were still in free-fall and though Royle had played me in every game, when Goat arrived, I could see Joe was building with next season in mind. We played together once in a 2-1 defeat to Bradford City, and we were very similar in our playing style. He was a great guy and would prove a fantastic signing, but there was no way we could both play regularly in the same team.

I was named on the bench for the next three games, by which time I'd seen that the writing was on the wall. I had a wife and son to look after now and the club were not keeping the promises that had been made to me, so I decided to take matters into my own hands.

I'd seen enough signs that my future lay elsewhere. I was aware of rumours that I didn't even want to play for City anymore, which couldn't have been further from the truth and really hurt at the time. I was available – if needed – in the final few games and had been having pain-killing injections for a number of weeks because of my ankle problem. My contract was due to expire in the summer and there was no security on the horizon for my family, so when my German agent Wolfgang Vöge informed me a Bundesliga club had shown a strong interest, I decided I wanted to know more.

I wondered if the fact I'd fallen out so publicly with Alan Ball had damaged my reputation? Perhaps some English clubs had me down as a trouble maker? If that was true, I wondered why they didn't canvass the opinion of the four other managers I'd worked under if that really was the case? But that's the way it was. It was time to put myself and my family first.

The interest from Germany came from Kaiserslautern manager Otto Rehhagel, who had watched me a couple of times and was keeping tabs on my situation. Eventually a private meeting was arranged near Manchester. As I was about to become available on a Bosman, talking to other teams was something I was entitled to do and had been since 1st January. Kaiserslautern were a newly-promoted Bundesliga side who were challenging for the title and in late April, Otto invited me over to Germany to talk more. Joe Royle had given us the day off so I flew back to Germany to continue talks – but didn't inform City. In truth, I hadn't made my mind up so I wanted to keep things quiet. I would tell the club when I had something concrete in place.

Cecilie travelled over with me because Otto liked potential new signings to be settled in their personal life and his own wife even sat in on our talks to give her opinion – he clearly trusted a woman's intuition more than his own! I agreed a three-year deal in principal with Kaiserslautern, and asked that they kept it confidential because of my situation at City. I was relaxed about the talks and we returned home.

The next day at training, Joe called me in. He asked me if I'd been back to Germany and I said I had. He asked if I'd talked to Kaiserslautern and I told him I had. He nodded and then told me to pack my stuff and leave because I was no longer a part of his plans for the remaining few games. He added that I was no longer part of the club as far as he was concerned, and also told me to keep away from the training ground.

He had always been honest and crystal clear with me, so I couldn't have asked for more clarity and I appreciated his directness. I had total respect for Joe but it was a sad end to a fantastic part of my life, though I had no beef with him and understood his reasons, even if I didn't agree with them. I had to do what was right for my family and Joe had to do what he believed was right for the team.

The truth was I was still totally committed to City and would be until the day I left. I knew I could have made a difference in those final few games. In fact, Georgi, who had also been left out, felt the same, yet we were out, in the cold and on our way out of the exit door. Georgi had agreed a £5.5m deal with Ajax and we went into our final game of the season needing to win and hope that results elsewhere went our way – exactly the same as it had been in 1995/96. But there would be one more ironic and cruel twist before the season was over.

We were playing Stoke City, who by now had moved to the Britannia Stadium, and they also needed to win to stay up. As I wasn't travelling with the squad, I got a ticket in the away end and sat with the City fans, hiding under my baseball cap initially before I was recognised. As usual, the supporters were fantastic with me and wanted to know why I wasn't playing. It was so frustrating because I was fit and raring to go – I'm not saying we would have avoided the drop, but I might have made a difference. We'll never know. Joe felt my heart was no longer in it but he couldn't have been more wrong. I would have done anything to have played some part in our survival. To me, it didn't make sense, but managers are paid to make these calls and they either live or die by them sometimes.

Of course, we won that game 5-2, but Portsmouth won their final game 3-1 to stay up while ourselves and Stoke were relegated. The irony was that the team who had relegated us was now managed by Alan Ball. He'd kept them up and had the last laugh over both City and Stoke, so all credit to him. Football sometimes conjures up the most incredible twists and turns – what were the chances of a scenario like that happening in any other sport?

Some people may question my loyalty but my situation demanded I took some sort of action. Besides, once I went out in front of the City fans that had believed in me and supported me from day one, I could never give less than my all. Nothing could ever have changed that because my blood ran blue.

If I'd been in Joe's position, would I have done the same thing? I don't know. It was a wrench to leave a club I'd wanted to finish my career at, especially as I'd been led to believe I would be staying for maybe another four years. I loved Manchester and the people who lived there; it was my home and I was settled, but that is the nature of football and being a footballer.

My main regret is that I never had the chance to thank our supporters properly. Georgi played the last few minutes of the match with Stoke and he did get the chance at the end to say goodbye, but I didn't. I think my record of 64 goals in 176 appearances stands up well and even though, after four-and-a-half years, I was no longer a City player, my relationship with the club and the fans didn't end there. Far from it – and they still had a major role to play in my life a little further along the line. They would always remain a big part of my life.

I said my goodbyes and told Georgi not to forget me, and to make sure I had two tickets to see Real Madrid whenever I wanted, because that's where I expected his talent to eventually lead him. He was that good.

So I was about to start a new chapter in my career. I wondered if I could reach the heights in the Bundesliga that I had always hoped I could, and maybe even force my way into the national team manager's thinking. Kaiserslautern had won the Bundesliga as a newly-promoted side, so I was off to join the champions of Germany so, in that sense, it was already looking like a good career move.

# 14

# Rückkehr nach Deutschland

## (Return to Germany)

Otto Rehhagel had tried to sign me earlier in my career on two separate occasions when he was Werder Bremen manager, and he told me he had been watching my career closely. I was a Bosman signing so hadn't cost him a penny and, at 29 years old, fitted his profile perfectly as I was arguably now at the peak of my career.

Money has never been my main motivation but I was unfortunate that during my contract negotiations, my German agent, Wolfgang Vöge, had been having difficulties with the tax authorities – an error on their part, not his – so when I sat down to negotiate a deal, he was unavailable and another representative from his office attended in his absence, who was maybe not as experienced as Wolfgang.

The structure of the deal was simple: a massive bonus when I played – the best money I'd ever earned – but when I wasn't playing, I would be on a very average income, particularly when you considered I'd arrived on a free and bearing in mind my achievements in England. But I read it, was advised the deal was okay and signed the papers. When my first season ended, it was a decision I would come to regret, but at that time, my mind was solely on the fresh challenge that I'd needed.

I'd always wanted one more crack at the Bundesliga, where I still felt I had unfinished business. My time in Nürnberg hadn't been a success and I still wanted to prove the doubters wrong in my home country. Kaiserslautern lies in the south west of Germany, close to the border with France. It's a small town surrounded by beautiful countryside and forests, but a little isolated. It's one of the main wine-making areas of Germany so there were a number of vineyards, too. All very pleasant and picturesque, and it didn't take us long to settle at all.

We initially moved into an apartment and soon felt at home, particularly at the club where I was reunited with two of the players I'd known from my days at the school of excellence in Leipzig. Olaf Marschall had played for Leipzig before moving to Austria with Admira Wacker. He'd then played for Dynamo Dresden before moving to Kaiserslautern in 1994, so his path had been not too dissimilar to mine. Jurgen Rische had been a couple of years younger than me but I'd played alongside him a number of times at Leipzig, so it was great to see them both again and we all got on really well.

We were all strikers competing against each other but it didn't

matter – we just supported one another and trained hard together, even though I knew if I didn't play, my wages would
be reduced by as much as two thirds. In Germany, and the
Bundesliga in particular, your pay is structured completely differently. I'd agreed a contract that was pretty standard for the
time – one third basic pay, one third appearance money and
one third was a win bonus, so you could have very good weeks
and in contrast, very bad ones.

If I didn't play, I'd lose 66% of my maximum pay packet so
it meant you trained like hell in order to try and make sure you
were in the starting XI. Otto Rehhagel played nine versus nine
or sometimes eight versus ten, and the training was often as
intense as a league game. On one hand, it kept players hungry
and the competition for places was fierce, but if things weren't
happening for you, your pocket would suffer. Having said that,
I only needed to play one minute off the bench to qualify for
my bonuses and Otto would always try and get you on.

In England, I always found I could never force my way into
a manager's thinking just by being good in training. I've seen
some players who took it easy in training and saved their effort
for matchdays – and the training wasn't so intense. But Germany was different and there were less midweek games to worry
about. When I'd been at Dresden and Nürnberg, the week was
always structured – Saturday to Saturday – with no matches in
between, so we trained really hard and you tended to see everyone else as a threat. That could have led to cliques and players
that weren't necessarily pulling together because of a system, in
effect, which meant it was every man playing for himself – but
Kaiserslautern was different.

The whole team pulled together as one and there was a good

mix and camaraderie in the dressing room. There were five or six of us, all from East Germany, who trained hard and got on really well with each other, among them, Andreas Reinke, the goalkeeper. I settled into the club far quicker than I'd imagined possible and I soon discovered that Otto Rehhagel was easily the best manager I'd ever played under. His man-management was superb, and he made players feel special. He'd work with you on an individual basis and help improve your game. For him it was really important to spend time with players whose squad numbers were 12-22, rather than those who were 1 to 11.

He was a master at the art of squad rotation, too, never doing it just for the sake of it, but to get the best out of a player to benefit the team. I don't know how he did it but he always seemed to get it spot on, too. He chose the right players for the right games – horses for courses, in other words. As an example, we played Werder Bremen and I scored twice in a 4-1 win, but I'd had a great chance of completing my hat-trick when he took me off 15 minutes from time. Inwardly I was seething but I didn't let it show – I'd learned my lessons – but then I thought that maybe it made sense as we had Benfica in the Champions League a few days later, and that he was probably saving me. It was around then that I learned trying to second-guess Otto was a waste of time.

Not only was I not included in the starting line-up against Benfica, I didn't even come off the bench! The next game, I was brought back into the team and had an absolute stinker in a 0-0 draw with Bayern Munich and I thought I'd be out for a while, bearing in mind the competition for places. Instead, I started the next game, too. He had his own logic and to have taken Kaiserslautern from 2.Bundesliga to the Bundesliga title in successive seasons was unheard of – this guy was right up there with the great mangers of German football and probably world football, too. His policy kept me and the lads on our toes, that was for sure.

He had guts, too. If were 2-0 down with 15 minutes to go, he'd throw on an extra three strikers and risk losing by a bigger margin in order to roll the dice – and we turned a number of games around by doing that. He just had a little extra – the X factor if you like. He managed to get the right chemistry in his team and he told me once: "I'm not going for the best players all the time; I'm going for players who function in my team and function in the group."

He called me, Olaf and Jurgen his East German school of excellence boys and always made a joke of it, but he knew we'd stick by one another even if one or two of us weren't playing and that, in my book, was clever management.

There was an incredible team spirit and togetherness and he pulled everything together – it showed out on the pitch, too, where we were again having a good season. Bayern Munich quickly started to run away with it and I think Kaiserslautern had caught everyone by surprise that first year, but we were holding our own and with 10 games gone, we were fourth and had already beaten Benfica and PSV Eindhoven in our Champions League group. A fairytale story was unfolding at the club, and we didn't know how high we could go together.

We had an unbelievable home stadium, too, and every week there would be 45,000 fans packed into the Fritz-Walter Stadion, so it was a vibrant, upwardly mobile club in every sense.

Then came one of my proudest moments as we took on HJK Helsinki in our Champions League group. I would have been happy to have stayed on at City and tried to help them out of the third tier, but the club had never given me the contract I'd needed to end my playing days there, so to play in the Champions League was a more than acceptable compensation. This would be a night I would treasure for the rest of my career in football as I scored a hat-trick against the Finnish side in a 4-1 victory. Okay, it wasn't Real Madrid, but it's nice to be able to remember hitting three in a competition every player in Europe wants to be involved in.

We progressed past the group stage and into the quarter-finals, where I'd hoped to draw Manchester United and get one over on them for the City fans, but instead we drew Bayern Munich and were comprehensively beaten over two legs. It was disappointing but we had still had a good run and could hold our heads up high. Ultimately, it had proved an enjoyable season and the move back to Germany had come at the right time. We just missed out on a place in the Champions League again, losing fourth spot on the final day of the season, and instead having to settle for the UEFA Cup. I'd played in about 90 per cent of the games and had finished as second top scorer. With two years on my deal to go, I imagined I would be finishing my career with Kaiserslautern. I felt I'd finally proved myself in my own country at the highest level.

I'd been really well rewarded for our season, with various payments kicking in for qualifying for Europe again; there were also appearance milestones and Champions League group stage progression – and these were big bonuses, so I had earned the most money of my career. Life was good, my family were happy and I was enjoying my football. I intended to kick on again for my second season at Kaiserslautern and was already looking forward to the new campaign. What I didn't expect was that one of the most disruptive 12 months of my career was to come, which would effectively leave me unemployed and heading back to England...

# 15

# Jeder für Tennis?

## (Anyone for Tennis?)

Our season had ended in early May and I'd been keeping in touch with some of the lads back at City, following the club's results all season. With City in the play-off final against Gillingham, I arranged to meet some friends in London and go to Wembley to cheer the lads on.

I'd always wanted to play at Wembley so this was the nearest I figured I'd get, so I flew back for the match and had a great day as a normal City fan. I met a few mates at the Hilton near Wembley and headed for the game. I was soon recognised by the supporters who came over in their numbers to say hello, shake my hand and sing my name – it was just like old times! My friends were amazed because they'd never seen anything like that before, but what else would you expect from City fans?

It was great to be back and I took my seat for one of the most dramatic games I'd ever seen, with City scoring twice in the last five minutes to force extra-time thanks to Paul Dickov's 95th-minute equaliser – if anyone deserved a moment like that at Wembley, it was him. City then went on to win on penalties and I think that was the turnaround for the club that helped put them on the road to where they are today.

I was just happy I'd been there to witness it all, though maybe a little sad that I hadn't been part of it. I met the players in their hotel reception afterwards and had a few beers with them, before they set off for their official reception. There was so much happiness, from the lads, their relatives through to the fans. It was a great day and I then went out to celebrate with my own friends before heading back to Germany for the summer.

My form back home had attracted interest from a number of German clubs because I was second top scorer behind Olaf Marschall, who was also a German international, but I had no intention of leaving Kaiserslautern. I was approaching 30 and we had just moved into a new house, plus Cecilie was pregnant again, so everything was moving in the right direction.

But as so often happens when a team punches above their weight, suddenly the hierarchy wants even more and they were determined to take the club to the 'next level'. Instead of sticking with the team that won the title and qualified for the UEFA Cup the following year, they decided to bring in some bigger names with price tags to match. They weren't looking to bring in say a Uwe Rosler on a free, they instead signed Swedish international Jörgen Pettersson, Youri Djorkaeff and Igli Tare for huge money. They were all strikers, too. I found it unbelievable because we had a strong group of players who had proved what we were capable of and had the harmony and camaraderie to go and kick on again. Plus, one thing we'd done the previous season was score goals – we might have conceded too many, but there was no problem with the front line.

I was confident I could hold my own, but with the contract I was on, unless I was scoring every game, there was no way I would be playing as often as I had been. Subsequently, that would hit me in the pocket quite severely. As I've said many times, I've never been motivated by money – but there was a huge difference between basic pay and basic plus bonuses, and it was enough to be a cause of concern.

It was around the time that the new signings arrived that I was informed that Berliner Tennis Club Borussia were sniffing around, and had made an enquiry about my availability. I was surprised that a 2.Bundesliga club had made an approach but a little investigation revealed they were owned by a wealthy insurance company who had wanted to take a team with no history to speak of, or previous successes, and turn them into a force in German football. They had moved steadily up the leagues and now wanted a side capable of winning promotion to the top league. They wanted to be the first club owned by a company in the Bundesliga and they also wanted to be the first German club to move on to the stock market. They'd ploughed a lot of money into building a strong squad and had purchased several Bundesliga players already – now they wanted to add my name with the added carrot of me captaining the side.

On paper, it was a nice offer, but not one that held any particular interest for me. I was very happy where I was but Otto told me it was fine to speak with them out of courtesy, which I agreed to do. In many ways I wish I'd turned them down immediately because when I saw the contract Tennis were offering, it blew me away. I'd thought there was nothing they could say that would possibly interest me, but the deal they were offering was huge, and had the added attraction of a guaranteed wage every week whether I played or not. The deal was for three years, too, so if I broke my leg the first minute of my first game, I would get the same money regardless.

It was a unique situation for German football and also very tempting, as it offered my growing family financial security for the immediate and longer-term future. Despite all that, I still left the meeting with the Tennis officials fully intending to remain a Kaiserslautern player.

I'd never been in a situation like that before and as I was approaching 31, it seemed almost too good to be true. I decided to have a chat with Otto – who had become a sort of father figure to me – to have a heart-to-heart about everything. Kaiserslautern were having a VIP barbecue and family day at the stadium as a pre-season treat for the players, staff and family members out on the pitch. I caught up with Otto there and told him: "Gaffer, I don't want to go. As long as you tell me I will be playing, am a big part of your plans and that you don't want me to go, I will stay."

He said: "I don't want you to go, Uwe, but I can't guarantee you will play as often as last season, but you will play."

I handed him the offer Tennis had made me. "Okay, but that is the contract they have offered me." Otto began reading and raised his eyebrows as he scanned the Tennis offer. I added: "I want to stay here, but if you can just get me a bit more on my basic pay, take it away from my bonus payments, but I just want a little more guaranteed. If we can do that, I'll be happy."

Otto said: "Okay, I'll go and see the CEO." And he did, the same day. Apparently, the CEO opened his draw to examine my contract.

"But Rosler is one of our best paid players," the CEO said. "No, I'm sorry. We can't do anything."

It was true that if I played and we won, I was one of the top earners, but if I didn't play, I was one of the lowest paid players. It was a curious paradox and my own fault for agreeing to the contract in the first place, but I hadn't had the advice I'd needed at the time and now it was causing me problems.

Otto informed me of the decision. He reiterated that he would play me a lot, but he couldn't say for certain how many games that would be and for me, it was now becoming a problem.

"Tell me what to do, gaffer," I said. "Look at these numbers they've put before me. I've never had a contract offer like this in my life."

Otto took the contract again and read it briefly. "If I was you, I'd do it," he said solemnly. That's when I decided I would sign for Tennis Borussia. From a football point of view, it was a mistake, but with my age and the money on offer, it made sense. I was leaving behind a coach I had nothing but total respect for, fantastic supporters and a group of players I'd become very close to. It was a massive gamble and it was the first time I'd ever moved for financial reasons, but I had to put my family first and they came before everything else. I should have followed my gut instinct, which was to stay and fight for my place.

I think Kaiserslautern received about £2m for me, which wasn't a bad return, and all profit considering I'd arrived on a free, plus my age and realistically being at the wrong end of my career. It was to mean more upheaval for us as we'd made friends and settled in the area, and I'd miss the calming, tranquil private life Cecilie, Tony and I had enjoyed.

I needed to clear my head and look at the positives – I owed that to Tennis if they were going to put so much faith in me. We'd be living in Berlin, which was a good base to be in, particularly as I'd soon be looking at moving into coaching. It would also be close to my family and friends, so it wasn't all bad.

I'd always thought that I would finish playing at around 33 or 34 because I needed that extra yard of speed to be at my most effective, and by that time, it would probably have gone. Players in their mid-thirties playing in the Bundesliga were few and far between in the early-1990s, too. It was rare because footballers didn't know how to look after their bodies and prolong their careers whereas today, there are a number of top players at the top level who are well into their thirties thanks to lifestyle changes, advances in sports science and nutrition experts.

So my thinking was that if I could help Tennis win promotion and have a couple more seasons in the Bundesliga, then hopefully I would have a chance of moving into the coaching side of things after hanging my boots up.

I'd enjoyed playing in front of the Westkurve during Kaiserslautern home games, where the club had the most amazing support. But even though I think they liked me, I never had the same rapport I'd had with the City fans – and I knew I would never have that kind of relationship again. Berlin was a great centre for football and I knew I could make things work using it as a base for Magdeburg, Dresden or Leipzig, where I was reasonably well connected and would have other options once my playing career had ended. Logistically and financially, the move made a lot of sense, but that's where logic ended, as I was about to discover.

# 16

# Spiel, Satz und Sieg

## (Game, set and match)

Sometimes in life you get a feeling that things aren't going to go well without any reasonable explanation – it's just a gut instinct, and from the first moment I drove into the Mommsenstadion, home of Tennis Borussia, I had bad vibes. I had driven to Berlin to sign my contract but still wasn't totally convinced I was doing the right thing.

The stadium didn't exactly inspire me, either. There was a running track around the pitch and small terracing that held around 15,000 people when full to capacity. It was a dilapidated ground with graffiti everywhere and, if I'm honest, it was a dump. There was no magical feeling that I had when I first looked around City or Kaiserslautern's ground, just a hollow emptiness. I thought to myself, 'What the hell am I doing here?'

I'd never played against Tennis before and I'd never seen them play on TV so I had no idea what the stadium was going to be like. I suppose, if I had I done a bit of research or maybe driven to Berlin before I made my final decision, I think I would have probably turned them down, but I was committed to moving now and I had to look past the stadium and see the bigger picture, which was why I was joining a project that could make Bundesliga history.

The manager, Winfried Schafer, had been part of the reason I was taking this gamble. He had managed Karlsruher SC for 12 years and during that time he'd built the club up and was a highly respected figure in German football. He had sold the club's ambitions to me, and I trusted his judgement.

He had signed a number of good players but while Otto Rehhagel's team ethics had been based on having the right chemistry on the pitch and a good blend off it, Schafer was completely the opposite and didn't put any emphasis on building a squad that would work together. He signed good individuals, but they were from all over Europe and Africa, all were brought in on massive wages – including me. I could see problems ahead.

None of us had ever earned this kind of money and it wasn't long before a few of them went off the rails. They didn't know how to handle their new-found wealth and I remember driving into the car park at the training ground a few weeks into my time there and looking at the cars that everyone had. Porsches, BMWs, top-of-the-range Mercedes – and this for a comparatively small 2.Bundesliga club.

I'd never been a captain before so I was on something of a learning curve myself, and I quickly realised we had big problems within our camp. There was a group of players who had brought the club up from the third tier to the second and these were good, solid footballers who knew the league – and there was another group of seven highly-paid players who had been brought in during the summer who were on perhaps triple the pay they were on. It was bound to breed resentment and it was a recipe for disaster.

So from day one there was a split in the camp. The manager, frankly, had no desire to heal the rift and I don't think he was particularly interested, either. He wanted me, as captain, to sort things out and so I got everyone together along with my vice-captain and worked as hard as I could to sort out the differences and jealously. Eventually, I told the manager he had to do more because we hadn't been properly integrated and there was no connection or camaraderie among the squad.

There were cliques all over the place and it was crazy. It was a massive challenge for me and there was huge pressure on us to win promotion at the first attempt, because the owners wanted a return for the fortunes they were paying some of the players. In spite of the issues, things began well enough and we were there or thereabouts going into the winter break in December. One point outside the promotion places, we were well placed to return in the New Year and hopefully kick on towards promotion. I'd managed eight goals in 19 games, which was an okay return – obviously I would have liked more – but things had gone better than I'd expected.

The squad went to La Manga after Christmas to prepare for the second half of the season and it was there, perhaps more than anywhere else, that I saw the unprofessionalism of some of my team-mates. To achieve our goals, we had to live, breathe and sleep football, but while football was still important to most of the lads, for some, so was having a good time and enjoying themselves. There were one or two occasions when individuals went out at night for a drink and they'd be drinking with players and coaches from other clubs as there would be a number of different teams there at that time of the year. They weren't even trying to hide what they were doing and, for me, it showed a blatant disregard for the manager and the club.

There was no discipline and I had to bring things to a head. I went to see Schafer and let him know that there was no way we'd be winning promotion unless we got our act together. I liked a drink with the lads as much as the next man, but there was a time and a place and this wasn't it.

I told him he needed to be firmer and he had to step in. He said: "No! That's your job. You and the senior players sort out the dressing room."

I told him the orders had to come from him, not his second or third in command. He had to lay down the law, tell us what was expected and what wouldn't be tolerated, and that we had to abide by those rules. Unfortunately, he wasn't capable of getting tough and that was the one weakness in his management.

So when we returned, the effects of the excessive lifestyle of some began to tell and we went on a terrible run that saw us go from fourth to 17th. The faster we fell, the worse the indiscipline became and as a result, the sporting director resigned in protest. We eventually survived the drop by one point. It had been a terrible second half of the season, but my warnings had been ignored.

I'd scored nine goals in 29 games and had a poor season by the standards I'd set myself. I'd spent too much time and energy trying to sort out the manager's problems, and I'd even handed the captaincy back before the end of what had been a terrible campaign. I'd wanted to concentrate on my own game again and though he tried to talk me out of it, I told him I'd had enough and that I just wanted to be a player again.

My second son, Colin, who I named after Colin Bell, had been born that year, so there was at least one happy memory, but as we went away for our family holiday in the summer, I was dreading the next season because I could only see things getting worse.

What I wasn't aware of was that the owners' gamble of buying their way into the Bundesliga had no back-up plan. There was no Plan B, and the season had been a case of 'win or bust'. We would be looking at another expensive season with a team, many of whom were on huge wages, who may or may not scrape their way out of relegation. I should have known what was coming next.

I was enjoying a relaxing break with my wife and sons in Majorca when I received a call from the press officer at Tennis Borussia. He told me the club had gone bust and that all the players' contracts were no longer worth the paper they were written on. The owner of the insurance firm was under investigation for fraud, and the papers were full of the scandal that was making headline news across Germany.

Of course, the officials at the club claimed paperwork had gone missing and that they had applied for the license needed to operate in the 2.Bundesliga, but there was excuse after excuse and eventually the league tired of their antics and kicked the club out completely. It was the easy way out for the owners, who knew they had to find a way out of the mess they'd created, so it was better to go out of business and wash their hands of the club once and for all. I felt sorry for the lads who the club had meant something to and the loyal band of 6,000 or so supporters who had stuck by the club, because they had been used and their club had been made a mockery of. So I was suddenly technically unemployed with no wages, unsure of where I was going to end up – I'd gone from one extreme to the other.

Then I had a thought. During the Christmas break, we'd gone for a family holiday in Dubai and I discovered Glenn Hoddle was staying at the same hotel. I saw him after lunch one day and went across to say hello. I asked him if he remembered me from my time in England, which he had. We got chatting and I asked if he fancied a game of football tennis, which he did, and we ended up playing for every day of our stay, on the beach just after the sun had gone down. Glenn was technically brilliant and I was exhausted after each game because he'd have me running all over the court, putting the ball in the corners on either side, toying with me like a cat with a mouse. It was great for my fitness, but really hard in the Dubai heat. We enjoyed each other's company, having long chats about football and a beer or two when we'd finished.

I learned a lot during our talks, and Glenn had a great football philosophy. I suppose I was like a sponge, taking advice and learning from people like Frank Clark, Brian Horton, Otto Rehhagel and Glenn, with the plan to become a manager myself again one day. But right at that moment, I needed a plan to continue my playing career. I felt my time in Germany had exorcised one or two demons and I felt satisfied that I'd proved I could play for a top Bundesliga side, while the experience with Tennis had left a sour taste in my mouth. I decided I wanted to return to England and called my agent.

"Give Glenn Hoddle a call," I said, thinking there was no harm in at least trying. Fortunately, Glenn was looking for another striker and so was receptive to the idea. I was soon on my way to Southampton to discuss a possible move back to the Premiership. Apart from re-joining City, this was the best possible outcome for me, and as the plane crossed the English Channel, I felt the adrenaline starting to pump again.

# 17

# Saints oder Sünder?

## (Saints or Sinners?)

I chatted with Glenn over lunch in Southampton and he asked me whether I'd be happy with the position he had for me in mind. At that time, I think Southampton were the only side in the Premiership playing 4-3-3 and I told him I thought I could slot in that system with no problem. He wanted me to be the centre-forward in his team, so it was a fantastic move for me. After agreeing terms, Cecilie and the boys joined me and we moved to Chandlers Ford, a lovely area just outside the city. Claus Lundekvam was a neighbour – and Norwegian, so Cecilie immediately became friends with his wife, while Chris Marsden was also living nearby.

I was excited to play for Glenn's team and was really looking forward to the new season. To be back playing in England was an unexpected bonus that I thought I'd never have again. There was so much to look forward to because Glenn had been someone I had greatly admired as a player, and he was a huge name around the world, so I was intrigued to see how I would fit into his plans. They also had the technically brilliant Matt Le Tissier still playing for them, though Matt's career was winding down by the time I arrived, which was a pity as I'd have loved to have played alongside him in his heyday.

I arrived at the training ground for the first time, met the lads and was made to feel very welcome. I'd had a hernia operation a month or so before I arrived and had a decent pre-season, though I was maybe two or three weeks behind where I would have liked to be. I'd not really done any strengthening work and as a result, about five weeks into the season, I overloaded on the other side of my body and needed another hernia operation. It was bad timing on my part because James Beattie came in for me and scored 10 goals in 10 games. A run like that meant I was going to find it difficult to just waltz back into the starting line-up upon my return and after that Glenn used me mostly as an impact sub – I was no longer the main man.

I could live with that because I couldn't argue with Beattie's record. He was 22, English and had taken his chance whereas I had just turned 32 and was obviously coming towards the end of my career – though I wasn't ready to hang my boots up just yet. In the past, I wouldn't have taken being left out lightly and would probably have brought things to a head, but I was changing with age and besides, I continued to learn from Glenn, played football tennis often and had long chats with him about football – not the sort of things you do if you are pissed off with your manager!

I knew I could learn so much from him that would be of great use to me in the future and we talked about tactics, training and various systems – everything in fact – and I enjoyed every minute.

So I had my second operation in Germany and was ready to train again within a fortnight – it was unheard of in England, and Glenn even asked the physio to take a look at the scar to make sure I hadn't gone back to Germany for a short break, which made me laugh. He couldn't get over the fact I could kick a ball normally, or run without any problems and do a full session after just a fortnight. I was proving a fantastic advert for German medical techniques!

I enjoyed training with Le Tissier, but he rarely played. He was still capable of brilliance during a session and scored some unbelievable goals, but he was a little overweight. I'd go as far as saying I've never seen a better finisher than Matt, and he could strike a ball so sweetly that it wasn't hard to understand why the fans still worshipped him. The forward line was Marian Pahars, James Beattie and Kevin Davies, and Matt was no longer the beating heart of Southampton. Respectfully, Glenn was phasing him out.

I remember Glenn saying that when you reached 30, you had to train harder and wiser than ever before to just keep on the same level. If you didn't do that, football would catch up with you and while it had caught up with Matt on a physical level, it hadn't caught me yet and I was still a few steps in front.

I never had a close relationship with the Southampton fans, but I wouldn't have expected to. It was a normal player/fan relationship and no more. Injury had kept me out of the home game with City, but in March, I was unexpectedly called upon for the game at Maine Road. I hadn't imagined I would feature, but when James Beattie picked up an injury after 30 minutes, I came on as his replacement. It was a pleasant surprise and the City fans gave me a great reception as I ran on, which spurred me on to try harder because I wanted to show them I could still do the business. We won 1-0 on a sunny day and it was a strange feeling to play against City who I'd never wanted to play against, for obvious reasons, and our victory had pushed them even closer to relegation, which didn't sit easily with me.

I stayed in Manchester overnight and caught up with some old friends. It still felt like home but although I featured in a few more games that season, I knew my time in football – as a player – was gradually winding down, at least at the top level.

Just before the end of the season, I was temporarily put out of action, not by a bad tackle, not by a suspension – but by my wife! I was told I'd be starting against Manchester United at The Dell and I was really happy because I thought it was a chance to get one over on United – something that had become ingrained in my DNA. This was such a great chance to prove that I could still cut it against the best, and my wife made me a meal of scallops to celebrate. The only thing was, I got food poisoning from an undercooked or bad scallop and I ended up being out for four weeks!

Of course, I had no idea there was a problem until I started feeling unwell and started vomiting. The following day at training I felt really rough, but I didn't mention it to anyone. I had to play in that game against United. Even though I was getting progressively worse, I made it to the warm-up on the day of the match, but as I did a short set of sprints, I was in agony with stomach pains and I knew I wasn't going to be able to play. I threw up and was sweating profusely, and I told the boss I was ill. I think Glenn may have thought I just didn't want to play because of nerves or something, but I was taken home and had blood tests the next day, where it showed that I had food poisoning. We haven't had scallops since!

Southampton would finish 10th in the table, which was a great finish for a side who had been expected to struggle, and I went away for the summer with just one year of my contract left. During the close season, Glenn left for Tottenham – a call he couldn't refuse – and coach Stuart Gray was given the role as the new boss. I knew things were going to be different and wondered where, if at all, I'd fit in.

I trained hard over the summer and returned fitter and stronger than most of the other lads who'd taken it a little easier on the back of such a good season. I knew I had to hit the ground running if I was to impress the new manager and I was flying in the pre-season friendlies, where I scored five or six goals. Gray had no choice but to play me after such a productive spell, though I think he had intended to start with James Beattie. Our first few games were against Liverpool and Chelsea and I didn't find the net. I think that made it easy for Gray to drop me, even though I'd played pretty well. The bottom line was I hadn't scored, he didn't have faith in me and I'd given him a reason to bring Beattie back. I was disappointed, but I wasn't going to sulk about it.

I knew my time at the top was limited and I'd lost that yard of speed that was vital to my game. The double hernia operations had also made me weaker, so while I still felt I could do a decent job, it was now more likely to be at Championship level. I wasn't getting much action at Southampton, where I was playing reserve-team football or on the bench, which was no good to me at that stage of my career. So when Cardiff City and West Brom came in for me on loan in October, it was perfect timing. I ended up going to West Brom and was cover for the injured Jason Roberts. I joined the squad at their London hotel and manager Gary Megson told me I would be playing the following evening against Crystal Palace.

So the following morning I turned up expecting a light session, but instead, Gary got us together and told us we were to go with the fitness coach, run around the perimeter of the university pitches and the first 11 back would start the game later that evening! I thought he was joking but I could see within a few moments that the players knew he wasn't. We ran, ran and ran – for maybe 25 minutes – on the day of a game! I couldn't believe we were having such a draining session with a match in just a few hours' time.

In the warm-up at Selhurst Park, I was already having cramp and I wondered if I'd even make it to kick-off, but as it was, I lasted 70 minutes, set up the winning goal and then went off. In my next game, I scored the winner in a 1-0 win over Nottingham Forest at the Hawthorns, so things had started well for me and for the club.

Megson was a totally different type of manager to Glenn. He treated me very well and was very direct, so I had no problems at all with his style and methods. By the time I left, we'd won six out of seven matches and gone from 10th to second – not necessarily because of me, but I had played my part, so it had been an enjoyable loan spell. I would've liked to have stayed longer, but it wasn't to be.

I was still trying to win myself a contract somewhere – one

last deal that would see me through to the end of my career. Megson told me he would have liked me to stay but they already had a crowd favourite in Bob Taylor, who was still at the club and aged 34. He said he couldn't afford to have another striker at the wrong end of his career as well, so I accepted the situation and returned to Southampton.

In my absence, Gray had been sacked after an awful start to life at the new St Mary's Stadium and Gordon Strachan had come in. On my return, Strachan called me into his office. Megson had written a letter about me, saying what I'd done for his team, how I was around the dressing room and at training – all very complimentary. Strachan said: "I've got this letter from Gary Megson about you – do you want to read it?" I said I didn't. He nodded, tore it up and threw it in the bin while I stood there. I smiled. If I'd had any doubt about whether I might be in his plans or not, I certainly knew now. It was time to find a new club and with the January transfer window just a month away, I had the opportunity to get away fairly quickly.

The wind had been taken out of my sails in an instant but I didn't mind Strachan, who was honest and direct. I knew where I stood with him, which is as much as I could have asked for. He was a character, fiery and if I'm honest, I liked him. My first interaction with him had been in the dressing room when he said: "Christ, I've never seen so many fat arses in one room."

Straight away he changed our training regime and he concentrated on our fitness before anything else. Sessions were longer, harder and more intense and that was needed at that point. Results soon began to turn around and we gradually climbed away from the foot of the table.

I knew I'd play no more part in the first-team at Southampton, but at least I would be remembered by the fans for scoring the last goal at The Dell in a farewell friendly win over Brighton the previous season, and also the first Southampton goal at St Mary's Stadium against Athletic Bilbao at the start of my second year – two historic goals that, with the greatest respect, unfortunately meant more to the supporters than they had to me.

So with my prospects under Strachan at Southampton seemingly nil, I knew it was time to move on again. Being at West Brom had given me a taste for playing again, and I wanted more, so a move to a Championship club would have been perfect. However, for one reason or another, it just didn't happen and there were no offers on the table.

Then, out of the blue, I was handed the chance to return to Germany once again. I was ready to move on so I thought, why not? It made sense for a number of reasons. What was the worst that could happen?

# 18

# Alle Wege führen nach Norwegen

## (All roads lead to Norway)

I felt my time at the top was finished, and the fact I hadn't really been able to win back my first-team place at Southampton had confirmed what I'd suspected for several months. I'd lost that yard of pace that was so important to my game, and it wasn't going to return no matter how hard I tried. I was 33 and I now had two options – play at a lower level or hang up my boots. I wasn't really ready to retire, so I accepted an offer from 2.Bundesliga side Spielvereinigung Unterhaching to finish off the 2001/02 season back in Germany – after that I wasn't sure what would happen.

I thought I was good for two or three years at that level and then it would be a natural transition into coaching, which was an area that I was certain I would move into after playing. Unterhaching were based in Munich which, like Tennis Borussia Berlin before them, was an ideal base for any budding coach to be based. It was only four hours from my parents and the family support network we'd never had since the boys had been born, so Unterhaching ticked a lot of boxes.

They wanted me to help the younger players and I knew I'd have a senior role within the team and would play regularly, but it was going to be a big ask. Unterhaching were second-from-bottom and in free-fall considering they had been a Bundesliga side the season before, and had held their own against their more illustrious neighbours, Bayern Munich and 1860 Munich when finishing 10th in 1999/2000.

I cancelled my contract at Southampton and agreed a small pay-off, though only a fraction of what was owed. In retrospect, it was a silly thing to do because I cost myself a fair bit of money by being too honest, but I wanted to play football again. I had perhaps been a little naïve.

Moving to Unterhaching was a gamble because they were teetering on the brink of a second successive relegation and if they went down again, there may well have been no way back for me. I agreed an 18-month deal and it was a calculated risk on my part, but they had some good players who I was familiar with. I thought there was every chance we would beat the drop.

As it was, things went really well and I enjoyed my time with the club. I'd like to think I played my part in the remaining games and I scored five goals from 14 starts, but we lost our status as a 2.Bundesliga side as it seemed to me as though the authorities went out of their way to make sure Eintracht Frankfurt weren't relegated to the third tier. We lost our final game, which meant we finished fourth-from-bottom and therefore we were technically relegated – but there had still been hope because it looked as though Eintracht Frankfurt, who had been plagued by financial problems, looked likely to go under.

I went away for the summer looking forward to a fresh start and maybe even a promotion challenge back to the Bundesliga. I had no intention of leaving, and the club told me that we would definitely remain in 2.Bundesliga because Frankfurt had no chance of winning a licence to play at that level. Who were they trying to fool? Frankfurt is the capital of German football, so they didn't disappear off the radar altogether.

So we were relegated after all and the sizeable loss in revenue meant Haching could no longer afford to pay my wages – in some way, it was Tennis Borussia all over again and I wondered if somebody wasn't trying to tell me something, as I was left without a club yet again. I could have forced the issue and insisted the club honour my contract, but there wasn't too much point. They'd made it clear they wanted me off their books and I needed to think carefully about what I did next, as it could well be the final move of my career. I'd got back in my rhythm after six months of playing football regularly and felt fit and strong so retirement still wasn't on the agenda.

I had trained hard and played in several pre-season matches for Haching – and we achieved a number of impressive results. A well-respected coach, Wolfgang Frank, took over and he fought hard to keep me on because even though we'd be in 3.Bundesliga, he knew I could be a major influence in getting the club back up again. However, the board wouldn't sanction it which, given their projected reduction in revenue, probably made financial sense.

Then, from out of the blue, I received a phone call from Norway. It was Kare Ingebrigtsen, a former City player who was now working as an agent in Norway. He said he had heard I was available and wondered whether I'd be interested in a move to Lillestrom? Apparently they wanted to sign me, and Kare, knowing my wife was Norwegian, wondered if I could be tempted. Lillestrom was about 10 miles outside of Oslo where my wife's family lived.

When I'd been at Lokomotive Leipzig, I remembered being a ball-boy in a European tie against Lillestrom so I was aware of the club and the memory was a pleasant one. As a kid at the sports club, me and the others had no additional kit or training gear, so with Lillestrom based there for a few days, we started to collect the players' water bottles they left around the training pitches and near their accommodation block. All the ball-boys collected a Lillestrom bottle as a souvenir, so I always had a soft spot for the club.

I didn't want to go to Norway – but when Cecilie found out, she was really keen on the move. Once she heard the word 'Norway', that was it and I might as well have gone and packed our bags straight away! In fairness, we'd had an unstable few years of travelling around, moving from club to club. She'd never complained and let me get on with things, so I felt I owed her this move.

I hopped on a plane to Oslo, still doubting I would be joining Lillestrom but with the intention of at least having a look around and getting a feel for the club before making a final decision. The Norwegian national team was strong, but all their best players played abroad so it hadn't been on my radar at all.

I landed in Oslo and was then transferred straight on to a

smaller plane. Lillestrom's training camp was the destination, as they were on a mid-season break in the mountains. We landed in the middle of nowhere, where I was picked up by a driver and taken through a huge mountain range until we arrived at a barracks resembling a few prefabricated units similar to those on a building site – that's where the Lillestrom players were staying. There was nobody around because the manager had taken them out for a meal in a nearby village and I'd arrived a little late. But I got a feel for the place and what the club was about. I knew nothing about Norwegian football or what the standard was, so I'd be taking a gamble if I did go. At Haching I knew it would be 3.Bundesliga and that I'd be fine if I wanted to play at that level, but this was different.

I wondered if I was doing this for Cecilie rather than football decisions until I met Jan Aage Fjortoft, formerly of Swindon Town and Middlesbrough. I knew Jan from our days in the Bundesliga when I was at Kaiserslautern and he played for Eintracht Frankfurt. The second person I met was former Oldham Athletic and Leeds United defender Gunnar Halle, who I knew from my days in England and had always got along well with. I think it was Jan who recommended me, and who probably told Kare to contact me and see how the land lay. These were two, well-respected players and it gave me a good early impression of the club.

I joined the squad for training the next day and in the evening we had a friendly match, which I scored in. The training pitches were good and I enjoyed the style of football. It reminded me a lot of English football which had a competitive edge and was fast-paced, all of which I really enjoyed. I spoke with Arne Erlandsen, the Lillestrom coach, after the game and

I said it was 'a maybe' and that I had quite enjoyed my visit. I still wasn't committing so I flew back to Oslo to have a look around the training facilities and stadium, and I have to say I was impressed.

The Arasen Stadion was a newly-renovated arena with apartments, shops and restaurants built around the outside, with the arena on the inside. It held around 13,000 and had floodlights that retracted into the roof so as not to interfere with the flight path to the airport – all very functional and stylish. I went home to think things over and while we were settled as a family in Munich, and football-wise it would have been better to have stayed put, I knew I had to do this for Cecilie. She had never complained while we'd been moving from apartment to house to apartment and so on over the previous eight years, and I owed her this move. She had raised the kids pretty much on her own while I concentrated on my career, so a chance to be back among her family and friends with a support network for the first time, was too much to turn down.

I was sad to leave Wolfgang Frank behind because he believed in me so much and after Glenn Hoddle, he was perhaps the most influential coach of my career, even though I spent a relatively brief time with him. Borussia Dortmund coach Jurgen Klopp would later claim Frank had been the biggest influence of his career, which is quite a compliment. He was way ahead of his time and a pioneer in many ways, using a variety of tactics and methods that nobody else in Germany really did at that time. He played with a permanent back four and used zonal marking – nobody else did that back then – and it was a pity we had to part company because of non-football circumstances. I'd learned so much tactically from him, talked for hours about football and I would have loved to have maybe spent a whole season under him, but it wasn't to be. He'd treated me with a lot of respect and included me in a lot of things he didn't need to, so that was the only hard part about having to cut my ties with Haching.

So we packed our bags and headed to Norway on something of an adventure. I was joining just in time for the second part of the season and because I'd kept fit and in shape, I slotted into the team well and scored 10 goals in 11 games. We finished the season really strongly and I think he knew that with me, Gunnar Halle and Ríkharður Daðason, who had joined us from Stoke City, we were going to be a force to be reckoned with the following season.

We had a great balance between youth and experience and Arne Erlandsen felt we could win the title with the squad we had. Things had gone better than I could have hoped and I was feeling as good and as sharp as I had for a long time. Everything was so easy – we had family around us to help with the kids. The boys had settled into new schools and could speak Norwegian already, so we were really happy in every aspect our lives.

The season finished in October and then we had a long break through winter, before pre-season training began around the end of January. So we had three months to prepare for the new campaign – it was crazy. We had a nice long holiday in the mountains, then went back to Germany for a while and had a great time with my family. I was hungry for the new season to start and felt refreshed with my batteries fully recharged.

We trained every day and we had to train outdoors because only a few of the bigger clubs had indoor arenas at that time, so it meant that we alternated between Lillestrom and Oslo, which was a little warmer, when the weather was bad. Trust me, training in Norway in January is not much fun and some days I'd be on a clay training court with salts spread over the top in temperatures as low as -22, but it hardened you in many ways.

I explained to Arne that I needed additional training to stay at the top of my game and I was grateful he allowed me to do a number of exercises that enhanced my own personal fitness such as uphill sprints and resistance sprinting, with that involving a parachute. It was a little unorthodox for the Norwegian lads to see someone doing these extra sessions, but it was accepted and wasn't a problem. We stepped things up with two weeks in La Manga but I wasn't feeling myself, and one incident worried me because it was completely out of character.

We hadn't been there long and we had a nice light training session with a couple of simple competitive games, but to me, it felt as important as winning the World Cup. I've always been something of a hot-head but I wanted to win this game. When the club captain, Torgeir Bjarmann, lay down as a joke to stop me being able to cross the line with ball [I was in another zone mentally and wanted to win so much], I only saw him stopping me doing what I needed to do.

I began hammering the ball into him on the ground and I couldn't stop. I kept kicking and kicking and people were starting to watch, probably thinking I was crazy. By the time I'd finished he had blood all over his face and this was one of the nicest guys you could ever meet – a 35-year-old consummate professional we called Mr Lillestrom. I wondered later what the hell had been wrong with me. I apologised profusely afterwards, but it was by no means an isolated incident.

During another training session I was caught by Gunnar Halle and I lashed out at him – I was 34, he was 37, yet I was behaving like some out-of-control 18-year-old. Something wasn't right and in later years I wondered whether it was the start of my illness. Was my body changing and chemicals being released that affected my behaviour? All I knew at the time was that it was not me. In training I was a beast, but when I got home I could hardly move and things were far from normal.

We played in a tournament that, after beating AIK Stockholm, Helsingborgs and Rosenborg, we lost on penalties to Helsingborgs in the final. Then we played a friendly with Rubin Kazan – we beat them 4-0 and I scored three goals, after which they promptly put in a bid of £1.5m. Lillestrom accepted it straight away! I said thanks, but no thanks! We drew with Austria Vienna 2-2 and I scored another two, so I had a fantastic pre-season and in Norway, because there are long periods of inactivity, the media take the friendlies very seriously. Our form was such that they made us favourites for the league.

The first game of the season was just a week or so away, so we headed off to Marbella for some warm sun and to finalise plans for the new campaign. We then returned home feeling relaxed and ready for the challenge ahead. It was cold in Norway so it wasn't a complete surprise when I started with what I thought was a cold. I continued to train hard and put it down to going from a warm climate to a cold one. We played our final warm-up game against our rivals, Valerenga, in front of maybe 7,000 fans, but I felt and played terrible. The cough had got worse and I couldn't breathe properly, so I had to come off at half-time. The boss asked me what was wrong and I told him I couldn't continue. He told me I'd had a fantastic pre-season and what had happened?

"It's the centre of my chest," I told him. "I can't breathe."

"It's just the air conditions; you'll be fine next week."

I was given antibiotics and sent to the clinic where they tested my blood for a virus or infection but they couldn't find anything. I carried on training but I was so weak I knew there must be something they were missing. I'd never felt like that in my life before, but despite telling the boss I was unfit for the opening game, he insisted I had to play and named me in the starting line-up.

"Okay," I said, "but I can only stay in the middle and just about get into the box. I can't run so you have to tell the others what is going to happen."

He agreed and I played the full 90 minutes against Bodo Glimt, and even scored the winning goal, but I felt dreadful during and after the game. The boss said he would send me to see the club doctor in Oslo on Monday morning, to find out exactly what the problem was.

I travelled to Oslo and had more tests over the Monday and Tuesday. On the Wednesday it was Easter and in Norway, everybody stops working and goes to their cottages in the mountains. It's a massive public holiday and the country pretty much shuts down so I was sent for x-rays on the Tuesday just before the private clinic was due to close for the break. I had the x-rays and then waited...and waited. I was the last person in the clinic, other than a few members of staff. Then the doctor appeared and said they needed another x-ray. I was a little worried but I had a CT scan and then went back in the waiting area until the guy finally came back.

"You have to go to your doctor straight away," he said. "And I wish you good luck. You'll need it." Understandably, that's when I got very concerned. I still didn't know what the problem was, so I went home, called the doctor and he said he'd get back to me when he'd seen the results.

Gunnar came around. We changed the winter tyres on our cars to the summer tyres and were chatting about the next game. I wanted to take my mind off everything. I enjoyed Gunnar's company, and our families had become very close. Then, halfway through a tyre change, the doctor pulled up outside our house. He never visited anyone at home, so I prepared myself for bad news.

"Uwe," he said. "We have to talk…"

# 19

# Jemand anderes Leben

## (Somebody else's life)

I had cancer – non-Hodgkin's lymphoma, to be exact, and I had the equivalent of a 12.5cm tennis ball in my chest.

I was to go into hospital immediately, where all the top cancer specialists would be waiting to treat me with all leave cancelled. My immediate reaction was that I wanted to go to Germany to be treated, but my doctor said: "No, Uwe. You have to go in now otherwise you won't survive past Easter."

From believing I had a cold or a chest infection at worst, I was now being told that, as things stood, I had about a week to live and the magnitude of what I'd been told hit me like a sledge-hammer. I was terrified.

Cecilie had taken the kids out while the doctor explained things to me and I think she suspected something was very wrong. I can't imagine what she was thinking during those few hours. She is an amazingly strong person and when I told her what the doctor had said, she stayed calm, calmed me down and told me that we'd get through this together. The move to Norway meant that she would have her own support network to help her through while she helped me to focus. Had we been in England, it would have been much harder for her, so I was thankful of that at least.

I was in a state of shock, trying to deal with the situation but failing hopelessly. I was manic, confused and panicking but I knew I had to somehow pull myself together and face up to reality – there was no way I could even attempt to beat this unless I did. I needed to start chemotherapy immediately to have any chance at all. The one question I continually asked myself was: 'Why me?'

I didn't know which of the three types of cancer specific to my tumour I had, but I did know that two of them are deadly while the third is the most aggressive but curable if you catch it at the right time – provided it hadn't spread. The good news for me was that there was only one tumour, but to be certain of diagnosing it accurately, the doctors would need longer than the time we actually had. They would need to take a biopsy and study it at the lab but we just didn't have the luxury of time on my side. They told me they were 95 per cent sure, but there was a risk of giving me the wrong type of chemotherapy – it was a risk that had to be taken. The treatment had to start immediately or else... I had to sign a waiver saying I accepted the risk, which I did gladly – what other choice did I have?

# KNOCKING DOWN WALLS

The chemotherapy started immediately and after just two sessions, an MRI scan revealed that the tumour had shrunk considerably. It was encouraging but there was still a long way to go and in many ways, we were still playing Russian roulette. But it was a sign that they had guessed correctly – it was an educated guess, of course – so things couldn't have gone any better than they had.

I had needed my own focus to get through the next few months and I suppose I went a little crazy for a while and shut off the outside world in a manner of speaking. I was aware of the life I had, but I was staring down a long dark tunnel to the pin-prick of light at the far end. Cecilie was the only person who could lead me towards it. I had a goal and that was to play football again and that I'd be fit enough to return next season. The doctors encouraged me and played the game a little, telling me that an ice hockey player had gone through exactly the same treatment and had resumed his career afterwards which, of course, is what I needed to hear.

I didn't consider what the chemotherapy did to your body and the toll it would take. I only imagined myself returning with a clean bill of health and playing for Lillestrom again. I had a circle of treatment that saw me receive chemotherapy for a couple of days, then two or three rest days, then a few more days of treatment, then three days' rest and so on and then the first circle was over. After a break, the next circle would begin and that was the pattern until you'd received your full course.

I was a little unorthodox during that time, going to the gym while receiving treatment and hitting the exercise bikes and pushing myself – but I needed to do that. I had to focus on my goal because that was my way of dealing with it and with Cecilie, my rock alongside me, I was just about managing to keep on track. I was in denial, but you do what you have to. The doctors allowed me to train and for the first week, I pushed myself and my body was okay. I got a good sweat on, but it didn't last and the doctors must have secretly thought I was completely nuts.

I recall one day early on when I was in the clinic bed and I got a call from Mark Buckley, a friend in England. He said: "Listen, Uwe, listen…" and in the background I could hear the Manchester City fans singing my name loudly around the stadium. It was incredible and so uplifting to know that they were with me and willing me to get well, and I can't express how much that meant to me. If I had a bond to the club before, it became unbreakable at that moment and it's something I will never forget.

Cards and telegrams started to arrive from City fans, too, The cards and letters had been sent to the club and they in turn had forwarded them on to me. I read each and every one and have kept them to this day. It steeled my resolve to know that these fantastic people were with me and it gave me another goal to aim for in that I wanted to return to the City of Manchester Stadium and thank the fans myself by walking on to the pitch.

While the City fans' goodwill was from a distance, my amazing wife kept me going in Norway. Every day Cecilie found the strength to come in and see me, give me hope and build me up, and all the while she had two young sons to look after and the prospect of losing her husband. She did that twice a day and only later on would she tell me she had to compose herself for an hour in the car before she came in to see me, and then another hour before she saw the kids.

I was, and remain, a very lucky man to be blessed with this

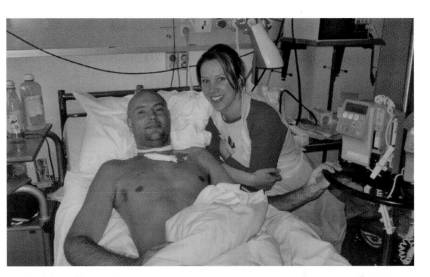

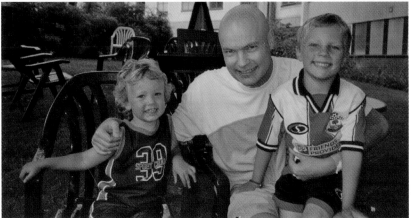

**Battling back:** (Top) In hospital in Oslo, Norway, recovering from cancer with my rock, wife Cecilie. (Above) At home with my sons, Colin and Tony

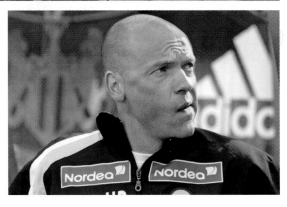

**Back in Toon:** Tasting European football with Lillestrøm, earning a 1-1 draw at Newcastle United in the Intertoto Cup in 2006

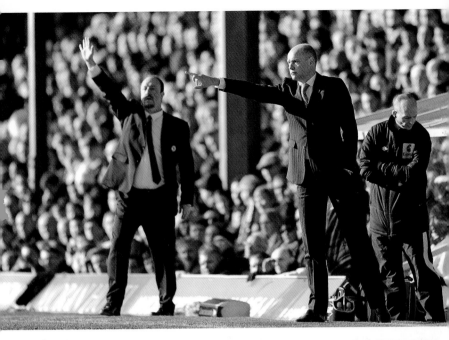

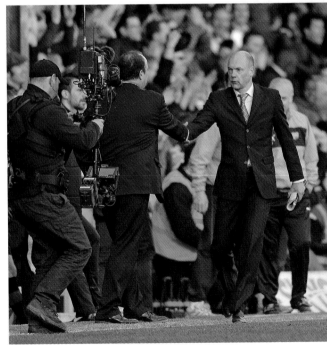

**Rivalling Rafa:** Scenes from Griffin Park as we came within nine minutes of what would have been a famous FA Cup victory over Chelsea, January 2013

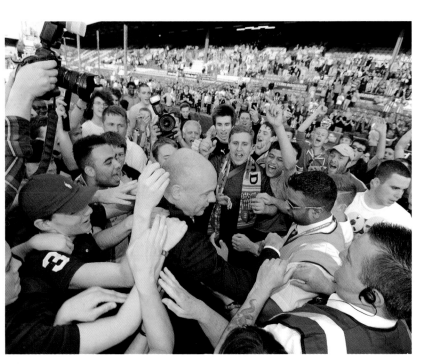

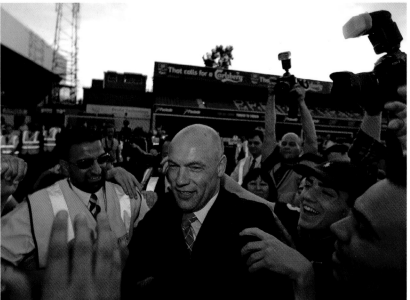

**Pitch perfect:** Being mobbed following our dramatic penalty shoot-out triumph over Swindon Town in the Play-Off semi-final at Griffin Park, May 2013

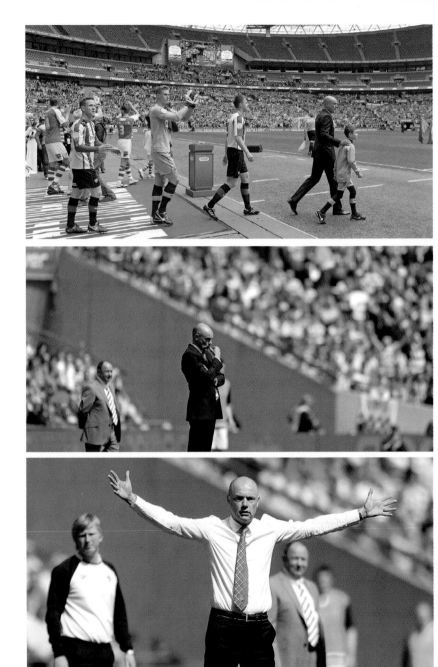

**Wembley woes:** The pre-match stroll onto the turf, replaced by Play-Off final frustration – Wembley is a lonely place for the defeated, May 2013

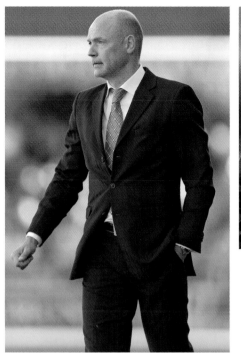

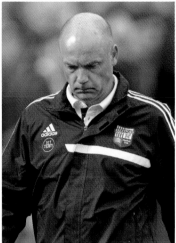

**Lost in thought:** The weight of the world on my shoulders following defeat to Bradford City, September 2013

**Suits You:** Watching on during the 2-0 victory at Coventry City, September 2013

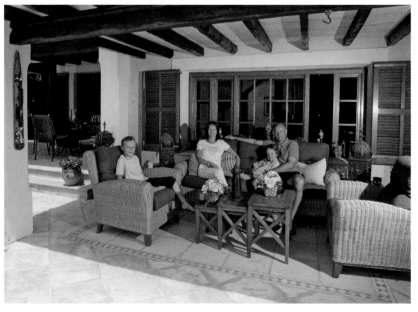

**Holiday home:** With Cecilie and the boys at our Majorcan holiday home

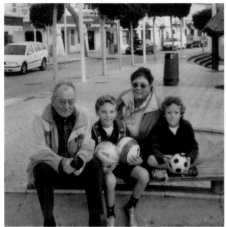
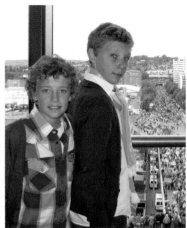

**Meeting the grandparents:** My parents, Horst and Ingrid, with Colin and Tony, and (above right) my sons at Wembley for the FA Cup final against Stoke City

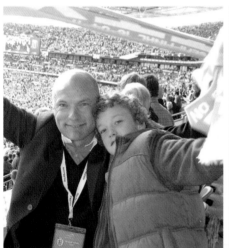

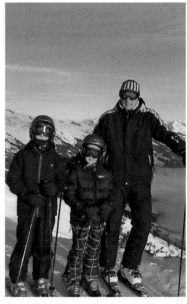

**Sunny scenes:** (Above left) Me and Colin at Wembley, and (above) skiing with my boys on holiday in Bad Gastein, Austria

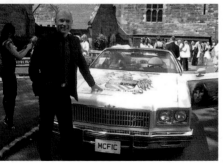

**City car:** (Left) At the wedding of our close friends, Gary and Angela Owen, in 2012

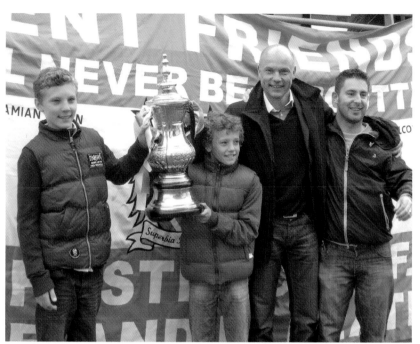

**FA Cup celebrations:** With my sons following Manchester City's triumph in 2011, and (below) with our good friends, Mike Pickering and Liam Gallagher post-match at Wembley

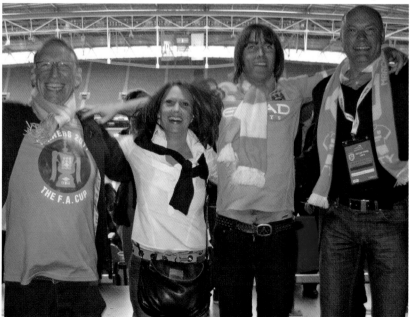

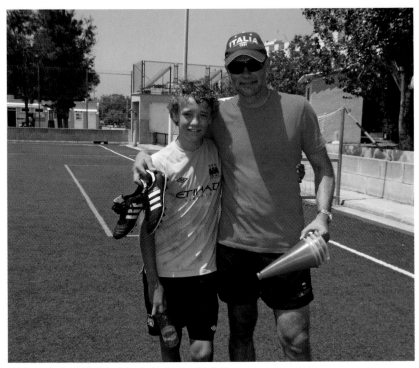

**Pitch perfect:** Football training in Mallorca with Colin

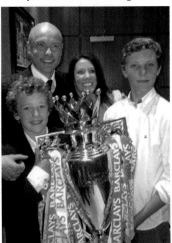

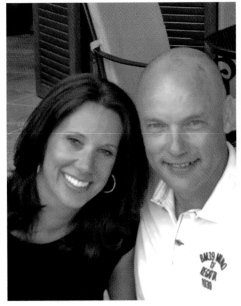

**Premier family:** With the Premier
League trophy after City's
dramatic success in 2012, and
(right) all smiles on holiday in
Mallorca with Cecilie, 2013

incredible woman by my side. She was always positive and never showed how worried she was, particularly since the doctors had told her privately that I only had a five per cent chance of survival. She knew all that, yet she was a tower of strength from the beginning to the end of this awful period on our lives. Destiny had brought us together all those years ago, and we'd overcome several major hurdles to be together. This was only going to make us even stronger.

Gunnar Halle was somebody else who was there for me continually throughout my treatment, and today he is like my brother. He had joined Lillestrom not long before I had and we'd become good friends. He'd been there the day I was told I had one week to live, and he came to see me every single day I was in the clinic, which for me was unbelievable. Prior to that, we'd been mates, but he drove in and came to talk football with me and he didn't need to do that. I will never forget the support he showed to me and my family.

Jan Aage Fjortoft was also a regular visitor and my Lillestrom team-mates began to visit when I think they'd come to terms with the situation. The manager was devastated, and the effect the news had on the club seemed obvious as they lost the first game since learning I was sick 5-1 to Molde. What had looked like a great season ahead was already fading and he had also lost his main striker with a life-threatening condition. I'd felt on top of the world and will never know how things might have gone. But the team's enthusiasm had gone, the team was deflated and all the momentum we'd built up in pre-season had been lost.

The treatment at least seemed to be working and my chances of survival grew with each passing week. Further tests confirmed that the cancer had not spread – it was just one huge tumour that was shrinking. I think the fact I was a professional sportsman with a strong immune system also helped enormously, too. My body had contained the cancer until the time I began receiving treatment, so I'd begun fighting before I was even diagnosed with the illness.

I had four circles of chemotherapy in total over a period of four months, with the first and fourth the hardest of all. The first session was three weeks long and is intended to shock your body; the second and third doses followed after a short recovery period in between, and the last session was known as 'high dose chemotherapy' and was the hardest of all because they want to make sure that they've got everything out of you.

I was told that if the cancer came back, that would be it. I had to remain in isolation for periods of time because your immune system basically shuts down and you are so weak and susceptible to illness that the slightest germ could prove fatal. I could see the kids and Cecilie, but only through a glass window without any contact because the risk of infection was too high.

It must have been so scary for the boys, who were aged six and three at the time and who didn't understand what was happening to dad. With each session I'd become weaker and weaker until it got to the stage that I couldn't even walk to the toilet – barely six feet away – anymore. My wife had to drag me to the shower because my energy levels were so low and even then I'd just sit there while she washed me. I'd need four hours' sleep afterwards because it had exhausted me so much.

The goal of returning next season had kept me going at the darker moments of the treatment, but I was starting to realise that I probably would never play competitive football again. I'd lost weight, had muscle wastage and was in pretty poor shape. After spending my whole life keeping fit, training hard and living right, I was now a shadow of my former self. But I wasn't about to let myself begin pining for my playing days – I had to be realistic. I was almost 35 years old, so I had enjoyed a good career and couldn't complain. I'd always wanted to be a coach so my focus shifted entirely towards the next chapter of my career. There was much to be done and above everything else, I was still alive. Even if I would never play football again, I could resume being a husband and father again.

Apparently, when my former team-mate, Michael Ballack, heard I was suffering with cancer, he said: "Uwe? He'll be fine. He's like a cat. He has nine lives."

After the past few months, I counted only eight lives now.

## 20

# In am tiefen Ende

## (In at the deep end)

I was feeling better. I was still weak, but I was starting to come out of what had been a nightmare. One thing you have plenty of time to do when you're in hospital is think. Although I wasn't ready to dive back into a normal life just yet, I had my new goal to aim for and with my prognosis good, it was no longer just a thought to cling to.

I called Arne Erlandsen and asked him what I could do to help while I recovered. He said he wanted me to analyse the games for him and then compile a report, so I began to study Lillestrom matches on DVDs from my hospital bed. Gunnar Halle had played in the games so he was a good point of reference for me. I told Gunnar I wouldn't be playing again but when my coaching career began, would he be my assistant-manager? It was all about visualising my future and whether Gunnar or Jan Aage Fjortoft, who also visited me on a regular basis, were just playing along with me I couldn't say. Psychologically, I was in another place and I don't think anyone would have wanted to take the wind out of my sails. Jan Aage smiled and said: "Okay, you're the manager, Gunnar is the assistant-manager and I'll be the sporting director – and we'll take over Lillestrom."

I said we couldn't do that. I would always be loyal to Arne Erlandsen and while he was in charge at Lillestrom, it wouldn't be a role I would pursue.

In between the third and fourth circle of treatment, I needed to have eight injections of chemotherapy in my spine, to make sure no cancer cells had travelled to my brain, after which I needed to remain perfectly still for four hours. The injection itself carried the risk of making you paralysed – a small chance – but again, it was always in your mind: what if?

I'd built up a close relationship with one doctor in particular, who I literally trusted with my life. He was one of the top guys at the clinic and he took me under his wing. He spent more time chatting and discussing this and that than he probably had time to. He specialised in the type of cancer I had and he took excellent care of me. I was quite a high-profile case with a lot of media attention, partly because top sportsmen rarely got cancer back then, so there was a lot of attention and interest from the general public. I got the best treatment possible and I wasn't on any private medical plan, just the equivalent of the Norwegian NHS.

So this doctor administered the first five injections in my spine without any hitches, but I would still need several more. He informed me his colleague would have to do it because he had to go to an international conference where he was lecturing, and there was no way he could get out of it. I told him he had to cancel because I didn't trust anyone else, but he told me he had to go and that I would be fine.

"Look Uwe, the doctor who will perform the procedure is as good as I am; there's nothing to worry about," he said, trying to reassure me, but I wasn't happy and it turned out with good reason, too. The day came for my injection and the other doctor came into my room, chatting with a trainee doctor from Pakistan, who was there to learn how to administer spinal injections. I almost did a double take as I saw my doctor had a plaster cast on his arm! He was talking the trainee through what would happen but didn't seem to be concentrating that much, and the fact I was there appeared to be incidental and no more. Finally, he said: "Okay, we're doing the spinal injection now Mr Rosler so just turn around, please..."

I looked at him stunned. "Are you sure? You have a plaster cast on your arm."

"Oh don't worry about that. I did it a while back and everything is fine now."

He was flippant to the point I thought he must really be good, so I turned over while he prepared to begin the procedure. "Just a moment, keep perfectly still..." I felt a scratch as he went in, but then he said: "Oh, sorry. I missed that time. Just a moment, I'll do it again..."

I couldn't believe what was happening. The slightest error could leave me unable to move for the rest of my life, and here was a doctor in a plaster cast, chatting away and not concentrating as he should have been. How could he undertake procedure that had dire consequences for the recipient if he made a mistake?

# KNOCKING DOWN WALLS

I shot around and told him in no uncertain terms he would not be touching me again and I told him to get out. I was absolutely furious and while he was very apologetic, he accepted the situation and left. A lady doctor came in shortly after because it needed to be done and couldn't be delayed for much longer.

Luckily there were no further problems. The other doctor returned and apologised again, and that incident was the only negative moment of what had otherwise been superb care from the medical team who saved my life. I can't ever thank them enough.

I survived the final high dose of chemotherapy – it can kill the weak and elderly – and with my treatments finally over, I still had one major procedure to go. My bone marrow, taken out before the chemotherapy, needed to be re-injected into my blood stream to give my body a kick-start and so regenerate cell growth and, as the doctor said, give me my life back.

There was a small chance that if it was rejected by my body that I'd die soon after, so it was yet another tense period as I awaited the results. There had been so many touch and go moments throughout my battle with cancer, but each time the best-case scenario for me had been the actual outcome. But the stress and psychological torment you suffered in-between was almost unbearable.

It had been an exhausting few months for my family and an experience I wouldn't wish on anybody, but I had come out of the other side and now it was time to move forward. Gradually, I began to regain some strength, though the first time I played in the garden with the kids I felt like an 80-year-old man. I could hardly walk or do anything, but I was starting to live again and life began to take on something like normality again.

Cecilie convinced me to either write a book or film a documentary during my battle with cancer, so I decided a film would be best with all profits going into a cancer research charity. I thought there would be interest in Norway, Germany and England so we began filming numerous moments during my treatment because I wanted to document everything I was going through. Later, an East German channel bought the rights, Norwegian TV showed some parts, but there was no interest in England. We would end up just covering our costs and raised no money for cancer research, but I was glad we did it because anyone who did see it would realise how important it was to have focus and goals to get through the treatment.

By September I was finished with the chemotherapy and I had a month off before I had three weeks of radiation therapy, which wasn't as hard as the chemo but was still very tiring. It never made me feel sick, which was something, and when it was complete, it represented the end of the treatment after six gruelling months.

My body was in a shocking condition. I was a trained sportsman and I'd never been in such poor condition so it was hard to take, even though I knew it wasn't a permanent state. Week by week, my energy started to come back and my mental and physical strength started to return. I rested a lot, watched a lot of football on TV and it was exactly what I'd needed.

By January, Arne Erlandsen invited me to return to the club for a trip to La Manga for the annual training camp and some warm sunshine. It was there I undertook my first training session with the strikers, which I enjoyed a great deal. I'd begun my coaching badges in Germany 12 months before and now I could continue along that road as I laid the foundations for my future. It was also good to be back among the lads again because I'd really missed the camaraderie and banter over the previous nine months or so. Fighting for my life in hospital meant that I was only ever with my wife, kids, friends and family, so it was good to get back to what I knew best. I enjoyed being part of a team fighting together, but throughout my battle with cancer, I had to fight alone.

The doctors had told me I should start to live a normal life again, and that there was no more medication needed. They advised me to eat normally, exercise and generally build myself up at a balanced pace. My body needed time to recover and all I would be required to do was have a follow-up in a month, then another two months later, then three months and then six months followed by one every 12 months for the next six years, after which I would be taken out of the programme and declared cured. It was a step-by-step process.

During my treatment, Lillestrom had initially cancelled my contract because I was unable to fulfil my playing commitments. It was something they were legally entitled to do, but the chairman, Per Mathisen, continued to pay me my normal wage throughout the final year of my contract. I had a special relationship with Per as he had signed me and helped my family when we moved to Norway. It was an amazing gesture by a very generous man, of whom I can't speak highly enough. The whole club had been amazing, and Lillestrom will always hold a special place in my heart because of the emotional rollercoaster I went on during my time there, though my association with them was far from over.

It was around this point that I received an invitation from City to fly to Manchester, stay in a hotel and then say hello to the supporters at half-time at the stadium, all expenses paid. I was very weak, and Cecilie and the boys both had flu, so we were all feeling under the weather, but I had to go because of all the support I'd had during my treatment. However, I wasn't really ready for such an emotionally and physically demanding trip. Cecilie had caught the bug off one of the kids and during the journey, I picked it up, too. I was lying in the Midland Hotel in Manchester not wanting to move or do anything. I had a fever because my immune system was still struggling to fight illness.

I couldn't let the City fans down though, so I rested as much as I could. I got myself ready the following day but I was shaking and sweating and not really up to it. I watched the first half and then walked out on to the pitch at half-time and the whole stadium gave me a standing ovation, which was incredible and once again, the supporters had given me a jump-start when I'd needed it most. I had needed to thank them personally and I wanted to show them that, yeah, I'd made it and what their messages and singing had helped me achieve.

I was too ill to attend a dinner in my honour that evening, and I instead went back to the hotel to sleep. We flew home the next day. I had to learn to pace myself and continue to build up my strength slowly, so I made sure I didn't pencil in any other engagements for a while. I'd needed that, though, and it gave me such a boost.

I knew my playing career was over so I needed to take a step back and detach myself a little. I needed to take up a more ob-servational role so I continued to build my fitness up and went to light training twice a week. In the summer, I continued my coaching badges back in Germany, and back in Norway there

had been some discussion as to who would be the next manager of Lillestrom. It had been announced that Arne Erlandsen
would be leaving at the end of the season – I'm not sure if he'd
just decided to move on or whether the club hadn't renewed his
contract. A few months before the end of the current season,
the speculation had begun as to who might take over.

At that point, I wasn't fit for purpose and was nowhere near
strong enough to take on such a stressful job, but I registered my
interest to the club through my agent, after I spoke with Arne. I
had total respect for him and told him that while he was in the
job or expressed a desire to continue at Lillestrom, I would not
apply. He confirmed he wanted to do something different after
several years with the club, and so I sent in my application to
become manager at Lillestrom.

I was shortlisted for the role and got an interview, but although I prepared myself as best I could, I was still very weak
and shaky during the process. I was under pressure because I
had to give a good account of myself as well as proving I was
physically and mentally up for the challenge. Looking back, it
was probably six months too soon to be subjecting myself to
that kind of stress. I did fairly well but they offered the post to
Stale Solbakken, who was also a former Lillestrom player (and
future Wolves manager), and they were keen to have somebody
who understood the club and what it meant to represent them.

Lillestrom occupies a special place in Norwegian football.
They have a reputation as a successful club historically and
were a team who were always hard to beat. If any team wanted to beat Lillestrom, they would have to work hard to do it
because it would often be a bruising, physical encounter, and
teams didn't like playing them. They are justly proud of that

reputation and while they aren't the most popular side in Norwegian football, they are respected and they wanted someone to continue an image that had been nurtured for many years.

Solbakken had an interesting background and had once been pronounced clinically dead after collapsing with a heart attack during a game, but thankfully he made a full recovery, retired as a player and moved into management. He knew Lillestrom well, had grown up in the area and was well respected within Norwegian football. He also had another advantage over me in that he had guided Norwegian side HamKam to promotion as a manager, so I'd always known the odds of me getting the post were slim.

It was a surprise, then, when Solbakken turned down the chance to manage Lillestrom for reasons that are still unclear to me – but the upshot was they offered me the job instead, which I was very happy to accept. I wasn't their first choice – I may not have even been their second choice – but I had no doubt I was their cheapest option. I didn't expect to become wealthy managing Lillestrom, but that's not why I took the post. This was a chance for me to kick-start my managerial career – a first step on the ladder – at a very well-run and highly respected Norwegian club. Arne Erlandsen had done a solid job and left strong foundations for me to build on, plus most of the players already knew me, so there was a degree of continuity. I had also been detached long enough to no longer be their team-mate or be too close to them. I'd purposely distanced myself in case this opportunity ever arose, and now it had. My appointment was officially announced in November 2004.

It was strange because all the discussions I'd had with Gunnar and Jan Aage around my hospital bed had now become reality with me in charge, Gunnar my number two and Jan Aage as the sporting director. Three former Lillestrom players in charge of running the club – it was an ideal scenario, and one that the supporters seemed very happy with. Now all we had to do was make everything come together on the pitch...

# 21

## Norwegian Blau

### (Norwegian Blue)

During my remission, Gunnar, Jan Aage and I had spoken at length about the players we wanted and the areas we felt we needed to strengthen – if we ever took over. We had effectively hit the ground running, the engine was already warm and we had a plan of action already in place, which was a massive help.

We had five months to prepare for the 2005 season, and our aim was to improve the club's fortunes after three successive seventh-place finishes. The club was having financial difficulties but there were still high expectations from the supporters, who believed the club should be finishing in the top three every year. I felt I could only benefit from taking the role on and had nothing to lose. I was a young coach at the start of my career so I carried no baggage with me, but I still had to make sure the shareholders and consortium who owned the club, led by Per Berg – a former Lillestrom player himself – were happy, not to mention the most important people of all – our fans.

Per Berg was the major shareholder who had bailed the club out financially, and had increasingly become more powerful as a result. I knew he would be watching my first season with a critical, knowing eye – not unlike anyone else in a similar position of power at any football club. He was no Roman Abramovich in that respect, but he had a major influence in everything the club did and he had the added extra of knowing the game inside out.

We had no money for transfers so could only bring in Bosman signings, one of which was German goalkeeper, Heinz Muller, who we brought in from Odd Grenland. He took some convincing, but he agreed to become part of our project. I was really pleased he did because he had Bundesliga experience and at 26, he was a great age for a keeper. We also added Michael Mifsud from Silema Wanderers in Malta – a striker who had played in the Bundesliga with Kaiserslautern – who was quick, stocky and unlike most Norwegian forwards.

We already had Robert Koren, who was my playmaker, so I felt we had a really good squad because Arne Erlandsen had assembled a very capable group of players over the previous few seasons. I just felt we needed a tweak here and there. I wanted to stamp my own authority on the team so while we would maintain the physicality, I wanted us to be technically good with a strong spine of Muller, Koren and Mifsud, and we would also bring in Kasey Wehrman, an Australian international who was a powerful defensive midfielder and a good passer. Bjorn Arne Riise would also join us, so even though Gunnar and I had no

experience in management and had never coached profession-
ally, I felt we had the tools to have a really good season. We'd
been thrown in at the deep end but we learned to swim quickly,
began the season well and had a good, solid campaign. In fact,
had we not stuttered in the last six matches when we won just
once, we could possibly have even won the title as we finished
just four points behind the champions, Valerenga.

I was learning, too. A few things I did in my early years in
Norway painted a picture of me that wasn't necessarily accu-
rate. I was new to management and not averse to trying different methods. I was probably a little outspoken at times, too.

A handful of examples might better explain why I was por-
trayed as, shall we say, a little different. Training on the Norwegian National Day was a big no-no. The day before was always
a big football day and then the good folk of Norway took to the
streets to celebrate. On one such occasion, we lost 6-2 at Ber-
gen the day before the holiday and I was absolutely fuming. We
returned to Lillestrom about 11.30pm, where I'd already told
our ground staff to prepare for a training session. We went to
our stadium where we couldn't put the floodlights on because
we didn't have permission from the airport authorities, so we
instead put the lamps on in the stand and trained under those
for one hour.

I then kept the players in the dressing room for two hours
where we dissected the defeat and cleared the air before finally
locking up and going home at about 4am. Of course, the press
got wind of what had happened and the die had been cast. I
told the media we had a game a few days later that we had to
prepare for and that I fully respected the National Day – but
I'm not sure they bought it! There was an outrage with ques-

tions asked of how I could do that and suchlike. It was an early lesson, but I was to discover times like that can stay with you for your whole career, so you have to be careful.

I was just different and I made mistakes, but the end result was that Lillestrom won four and drew two of their next six games. However, my image of being a little bit hot-headed and crazy at times followed me around like a hungry dog. I was different and unpredictable but Norwegians like to know where they are at with someone and, as a rule, are non-confrontational.

Another time we were away to Fredrikstad and we won 1-0, which was a great result because they were a tough nut to crack on their own ground. There were gale force winds blowing across the pitch that day and Norwegian grounds are usually more open than say those in England.

In the first half we couldn't get the ball outside of our own half and often, not even out of our own area. When our goalkeeper kicked it out, it would blow straight back towards us, but we dug in and knew that if we could reach half-time with the score 0-0, we'd have a great chance when we had the wind. Against the odds, we went in level at the break and when it was our turn to have the gale behind us, we got an early goal and then kept the ball because the match was as good as over.

Afterwards at the post-match press briefing, a lady journalist asked me a question that, frankly, got my back up a little. Bearing in mind the conditions and the game she'd just watched, she said: "Can you tell me why you totally underplayed in the first half?" That was not a good thing to say. I took the lady over to the window that looked out on to the pitch and, in front of the other journalists, pointed to the flags whipping in the wind on the stand opposite.

"Pardon me," I said, pointing. "I'm not being sexist, but that is the reason we didn't perform." I then walked away. For me it was sloppy journalism. I welcomed ladies working in football and I had no problem whatsoever with women taking up leading roles within the game. In my eyes this was about simple laziness, and not seeing the bigger picture. I suppose she just got my back up because I'd been so happy with our display and, to me, she displayed a lack of understanding. Had it been a man, I'd have done exactly the same thing.

The next morning, Cecilie was in the supermarket when she saw the front page of one of the national papers with the headline: 'Uwe Rosler: Male chauvinist'. I was flabbergasted. In England, nobody would think anything of it, but in Norway it was a national crisis that ended with me explaining myself to our owner, sporting director and, when I got home, Cecilie, who also gave me a hard time!

For a time, everything I did seemed to make headline news. There was yet another occasion when I was a little naïve. We were playing away to Odd Grenland, who were in the process of building a massive new stand behind our benches at the Skagerak Arena. As ever, I was always drinking loads of water and halfway through the second half, I got caught short and had to go to the toilet. It was bad luck for me that the toilets were in the stand opposite! I knew I'd never make it because I'd have to walk around the pitch.

I told Gunnar to take over for a moment while I sneaked to the back of the benches, where I kneeled down and took a sly pee. Little did I know that a camera was pointing at me so when the game finished and I shook the other manager's hand, the players, the referee and linesmen, the papers said I'd gone to the toilet but hadn't washed my hands. The press had a bit of fun with the story which made me smile if I'm honest, but it was yet another example of how eyes are always on you whatever you do when you're in the public eye!

Lesson, lessons, lessons…

So we finished in fourth place in that first season and qualified for the Scandinavian version of the Champions League, called 'The Royal League' – a competition pitting the top clubs of Sweden, Denmark and Norway against each other along the lines of the Champions League which, by November, most Scandinavian sides that had been involved would now have been eliminated from. It was a gap filler, but a lucrative one if you progressed to the latter stages. It was only the second year it had been held but it had a lot of money behind it and the sponsors were determined it would be a success. In many ways it was manna from heaven because it would run from November to April and meant the overly-long break we had to take during winter would not be a problem.

But first we had the Norwegian Football Cup Final to look forward to – Norway's version of the FA Cup – against Molde. It was the first time in 13 years that Lillestrom had reached the final and it was the chance to cap off a great first season. We went into extr-time level at 2-2, but ended up losing 4-2. I learned some lessons in that game where my inexperience showed as a new manager. I had tried to make our preparation perfect where in later years, I learned that you have to keep games like that as normal as you can. Molde had been fighting against relegation so we were clear favourites, but we just didn't turn up on the day.

The Royal League kicked off shortly after the season ended

and it was a fascinating challenge for me and the players. It would also provide some much-needed finance during a period when the club would traditionally have relatively little or no income. So there were no long holidays for the players this year and we drew Danish sides FC Copenhagen and Brondby, plus Swedes Kalmar – a really tough group.

Of course, the games were still being played in freezing conditions and the clubs had to heat the pitch throughout the competition – it wasn't uncommon to play in temperatures of minus 10 degrees. Valerenga wanted to play their games indoors so the structure wasn't ideal, and it wasn't easy to complete the fixtures. But we struggled on and won our group with two wins and four draws from six games.

We then beat IFK Gothenburg, now managed by good friend Arne Erlandsen, in the quarter-finals and Djurgardens in the semis to reach the final which was a massive achievement for us. The final, in Copenhagen, was against FC Copenhagen – where Stale Solbakken had literally just taken over – it was a small world!

We had already played in their home stadium, and had drawn home and away against them in the group stages so we knew we were, at worst, two evenly-matched teams. The final proved a tight game, but we lost to a solitary goal scored in stoppage time, which was obviously very disappointing. At least we'd flown the flag for Norway because the Danes and Swedes traditionally looked down on Norwegian football, comparing us to farmers and country bumpkins. But we'd matched the best Scandinavia could produce and the lads could hold their head high.

What the Royal League had given us was fantastic preparation for the new season because we'd been playing competitive football throughout the winter, whereas most of our opponents hadn't, so we felt more confident than ever. As a club, we were also more financially stable than we had been for many years. Lillestrom were losing around 16m Krone a year and in one season we had actually balanced the books by breaking even thanks to a good domestic campaign, the cup final and the Royal League final appearances plus TV revenue and additional gate money and bonuses.

So despite all the good things that had happened, I was a little dismayed that Per Berg still seemed to doubt me as a manager. He was critical on occasion and I felt he didn't have complete faith in me – I had no idea why, and thought two finals and a top-four finish was reason enough to believe that I had been a good choice for manager. It had been one of Lillestrom's best and most exciting campaigns for many years, but there was still something not quite right.

I'd been a popular choice with the supporters but I felt Per believed that it was a win-win situation because if I failed, the cost would be minimal to sack me whereas if things worked out, it would reflect well on his judgement. He at least backed me in the transfer market though, as we added a young Canadian striker to the squad – Olivier Occéan – at a cost of 7m Krone – our first big purchase for some time.

Again we started well and, as one of the favourites for the title, we led the table for the opening few months of the campaign. But I was constantly having to answer questions from Per Berg, who wanted to know why we were doing this, that and the other. The reason, I discovered eventually, was that Per wanted to bring in Tom Lund, considered Norway's greatest-ever player and someone who had been compared to Johan Cruyff during an illustrious playing career, as his new manager. Tom was a national hero and a former Lillestrom player, but he was also someone Berg regularly went to for advice. Tom was somewhat pushed on to me for discussions on tactics, training and selection, but I really bought into it because he was a good guy and very knowledgeable. I don't think Tom felt comfortable with the role because he didn't want to step on my toes or be seen as too influential. In fact, because he was shy and respectful, he probably held himself back a little and the owner believed that was solely down to my personality and that I was resisting his help. Nobody said that, but that was how I felt.

Jan Aage explained that Gunnar and I were anything but resentful of Tom's involvement, but it got to the stage when Per wanted Tom to take one or two training sessions a week and I said that would never happen while I was manager. We'd been going along really well and there had been no problems, but suddenly I was being put in a situation that was making my position untenable. Per clearly didn't trust me to run his team and it was reaching the stage where we were both uncomfortable with the way things were going, which had a negative impact on our season. I was the manager and therefore expendable whereas he held the purse strings and the club relied on his money to survive. How could I possibly win?

At least the Intertoto Cup provided a welcome distraction. We had drawn Newcastle United and I relished the challenge of facing a Premiership club and returning to England again – though I forgot my passport on the outgoing journey, missed the flight and one training session and then arrived just in time for the press conference the next day! Our fans were excited as well because of their love of English football – this was an all-too rare opportunity to pit our wits against a fantastic and famous football club.

We played in July 2006 and we felt we could give it a real go, particularly as Newcastle were fresh from pre-season. The first leg was at St James' Park in front of more than 31,000 people and we were superb, taking the lead through Robert Koren. They equalised through Albert Luque but we had taken on a side packed with quality players such as Shay Given, Nolberto Solano, Shola Ameobi, James Milner, Emre and Scott Parker, and left the pitch to a standing ovation from the home fans after a thoroughly deserved 1-1 draw. We had the away goal and a real chance of progressing to the UEFA Cup, but I think they learned their lesson, came to Norway four days early to prepare and won 3-0 at our place. However, we'd done ourselves no harm and represented Norway with great pride.

Domestically, our form had dipped and I spent a lot of time fighting battles that I shouldn't have had to and ended up fighting my corner in board meetings, arguing with Per Berg and expending a lot of energy, which should never have happened. There are better ways to defend one's self but I was still on a learning curve. We'd dropped to third in the table and the situation reached a head when I said I could no longer work under the conditions being imposed on me.

I told Per if he didn't trust me, he should get in someone that he did. He responded by saying that's exactly what he would do. I suppose I'd given him the chance to call my bluff, and he had. We completed the season and once again finished fourth, though this time, after the start we'd had, we probably should have finished in the top three.

I felt one of the main reasons we'd lost our way a little was down to the fact we'd lost one of our best players, a Swedish wing-back called Christoffer Andersson – who formed part of a really strong right flank – midway through the season. He had six months of his contract remaining when Hannover came in for him and I told the board that if we sold him, we were selling the championship because he was our best attacking threat, a set-piece specialist and an integral part of the team. They didn't listen and he headed off to the Bundesliga at a cost of 4m Krone. We subsequently suffered, as I knew we would. We then brought in a right-back from Brondby, who was nowhere near fit. We couldn't find a short-term replacement who was anywhere near as effective, but there was nothing I could do.

Our Royal League participation meant we hadn't had a break for 18 months. The players became mentally tired towards the end of the season so that had come back to bite us, too, as we had a relatively small squad. Norwegian players simply weren't used to playing so many games. Even going into the final month of the season we were still in with a good chance of winning the title but lost some games we should not have had done in the run-in. Per and I were cold towards each other and I still think if we'd had a good working relationship, we would probably have won the title.

On the afternoon before the final game of the season – and with plenty still at stake – I received a phone call to inform me that Per Berg had met with another manager to discuss replacing me. I knew my time at Lillestrom was coming to an end and I was absolutely fuming. I was told I would be replaced after the match but I had to look after my players first and foremost as there was still a game to play. We finished with a 2-0 victory over Henning Berg's Lyn Oslo, but results elsewhere didn't go our way and we finished fourth again. It had been an acceptable season and the Lillestrom supporters still seemed very happy, but my time there was over.

Viking boss Tom Nordlie had been lined up but I still flew out with my coaching staff to my home in Majorca for a few days of sunshine and golf. I hadn't heard anything official yet, but it was only a matter of time and not long after the plane landed, I received a call from Jan Aage Fjortoft. He had always fought for me at board level and I knew he wanted the best for me and the football club. I trusted him implicitly.

"Come into work on Monday and both you and Gunnar prepare yourself for the worst," Jan Aage told me as I finished a nice relaxing meal. It was confirmation of what I already knew to be inevitable.

I told him I'd be there and on my return, I went to the stadium where the lads were in for training. I said my goodbyes to the players which was a very emotional moment for me. Some of them were crying and I had tears in my eyes, but it was time to move on. I walked from the dressing room, around the pitch and towards the offices where my contract would be cancelled and a statement would be read out to the waiting media. On that short walk, Jan Aage joined me and said: "The next 10 minutes will decide your future as a manager, Uwe..."

I knew he meant that my reaction and behaviour at the press conference would determine how I was perceived by prospective employers and Jan Aage, as usual, was spot on. If I let my emotions bubble to the surface, I'd probably be looked upon as some sort of volatile character that had brought this situation on himself. I must admit, there had been every chance I would have reacted exactly that way. I was feeling emotional and felt

I'd been poorly treated.

"Be professional, bite your lip and be calm – or say what you want to say and you will probably find it difficult to find work again," he added. "So you decide what you want to do, Uwe."

I had so much anger in me that but for Jan Aage's intervention, I'd almost certainly have let Per Berg have both barrels at the press conference. Instead, I didn't say anything untoward, composed myself and was professional from start to finish. I said that I didn't agree with the decision but that I accepted it. I wished the club all the best and said that now I would move on.

It was probably the best piece of advice I'd ever received from a very close friend and afterwards, Jan Aage expressed his own dissatisfaction with the decision to replace me by making it clear it was nothing to do with him, and that he didn't agree with the board on this occasion. It was a shock, and I don't think I deserved to be moved on, but within a week I would be back in a job, proving Jan Aage's press conference theory to be spot-on.

# 22

## Die Wikinger kommen

### (The Vikings are coming)

Just six days after being dismissed from Lillestrom, Viking Stavanger were on the phone offering me a new job. My head was spinning as I was still trying to understand the events of the previous few days, so this came completely out of the blue, but with a slightly bitter aftertaste from my first managerial role, I thought there was no better thing to do than to jump right back on the bike I'd just fallen off and start pedalling again.

Viking were one of the biggest clubs in the country but I couldn't help but wonder what might have happened had I been allowed to continue at Lillestrom because we'd been building something special there with a lot of very good young players, a great team spirit and good work ethic. Yes we would have needed to fine-tune one or two things and freshen up everything from staff to training and tactics, but these were minor issues and part and parcel of running a football club. I didn't say a bad word about the club or the owner after my departure and let others do the talking for me.

Per Berg received a lot of criticism for sacking me and Gunnar from the media – and from the Lillestrom fans, who hadn't seen my dismissal coming. The truth was Berg had wanted a more experienced man at the helm because he thought they could take the club to another level. He gave the new man a lot of money to spend and they again finished fourth the following season, though in fairness, they did at least win the Norwegian Cup. Thereafter, the team went into a steady decline, never even finishing above 10th position for the next four seasons, which was shame because they had great supporters and there were some very good people at the club. I think it's probably fair to say the expectation levels among the fans and media have also fallen somewhat over the past few years, but that gives me no pleasure.

I had a new challenge in front of me and Lillestrom were now part of my past, though the club will always have a special place in my heart. I finished my playing career with them and starting my management career there, too. Plus, I'll never forget the way Per Matthisen looked after me and my family when I was ill so I wish them only well.

As a footnote to this part of my life, in 2013 Jan Aage invited me to watch Arsenal v Liverpool at the Emirates Stadium with a group of sponsors from Norway – and among the party was Per Berg. We had a nice dinner and talked about the past and everything is okay between us. Time, as they say, is a great healer.

Viking had avoided relegation on the final day of the season after winning their last game and staying up on goal difference. The irony of their vacant managerial position was that Tom Nordlie had left Viking to take over at Lillestrom so we were, in effect, swapping jobs. Nordlie had only taken over Viking on a short-term contract and had done well there, but I believe Lillestrom had contacted him during his spell to sound him out about replacing me. The managerial merry-go-round, I believe it's called.

I wanted to get back into football straight away and Gunnar came with me as my right-hand man. The only problem Cecilie and I had was that we'd only just moved into our dream home near Lillestrom. Cecilie had put so much into the project that it was a real wrench to leave. When I'd finished my cancer treatment and the prognosis had been confirmed as very positive, we'd decided, as a family, to build our own home as we'd been renting before that. We wanted to put down our roots there because it was close to Cecilie's family, plus Oslo was close by and the airport was just a short drive away, too.

We found a beautiful plot of land, high up on a hillside overlooking a valley and purchased it, though we were initially refused building permission by the local authority. It was the only place we wanted to live and because it was an established area, there were no other options available. We were told by various people that because the high speed train ran in a tunnel far beneath the land, building directly above it was impossible.

Cecilie knew football would take the majority of my time up so she began to ask questions to the relevant authorities about why we couldn't build there and when she finally got to the people who made the decisions, they told her that as long as some minor building specifications were followed, the building work would be fine to get the go ahead. Everything we'd been told had merely been assumption and rumour. Cecilie went from the owner to his lawyers to the government and it was her determination that allowed us to continue with our plans. Cecilie led the whole project from start to finish, as I'd just taken over at Lillestrom and she saw the whole project through. But we'd lived there just a few months when I got the sack!

Stavanger was on the west coast of Norway and an hour's flight from Oslo, so I couldn't commute by car which meant we had to move to Stavanger and leave our beautiful new home behind. The house would stand empty for nearly two years before we sold it, having never really lived there, which was a great shame considering all the time and effort Cecilie had put in. Unfortunately, that is one of the downsides of a life in football, where it's a case of wherever you lay your hat, that's your home.

So we bought a three-bedroom apartment by the sea which was beautiful, and we found Stavanger a really nice place to live. Viking had a new stadium, were financially sound and one of the major forces in Norwegian football, even if they had lost their way a little in recent times. I inherited an experienced squad and one that had the capability do far better than it had done in recent seasons, so I felt confident we could make some excellent progress in the months ahead. Former Southampton, Blackburn and City (briefly) striker Egil Ostenstad was the sporting director at Viking, where he had attained legendary status during two successful spells with the club.

# KNOCKING DOWN WALLS

We had a terrific first season, though we endured a difficult start – perhaps a hangover from the previous season – winning just one of our opening six games. My first trip back to Lillestrom came in that opening spell and we went down 4-1, but things steadily improved thereafter and we made the Viking Stadion a fortress, remaining unbeaten all season and eventually finishing third – one place above Lillestrom – the club's highest finish since 2001.

It had been an enjoyable first year in Stavanger, but I found that it was quite an intense place to manage a club. Due to it being isolated on the west coast, it is the main focus of the people who live there and the majority eat, breathe and sleep Viking. Being the main headquarters for Norwegian oil and gas companies, it was also one of the richest cities I've ever been to and the standard of living was very high. There was so much wealth and the infrastructure and schools were as good as you would find anywhere. Even our brand new 16,300 capacity stadium had heaters built into the roof to blow warm air down and keep our fans warm – it was unbelievable.

We probably overachieved massively in that first season and played some great, attractive football in the process. We had a Nigerian striker called Peter Ijeh who scored 18 goals in 23 games, and I had proved again that I could improve teams within a short space of time. At Lillestrom I'd taken over a team that was a solid mid-table side and gradually improved their fortunes, but this was side with a lot of foreign players, very experienced with their own opinions and yet we'd gone from third-bottom to third-top in the space of 12 months, so there was a lot to be pleased about. There were three Danish internationals, three Swedes and a few players from African countries in the squad as well as a strong core of Norwegians. A few years earlier they had also been managed by Roy Hodgson.

The players were far more vocal than they had been at Lillestrom, but I put that down to the fact we had 10 players who were either over 30 or approaching that age. It was a completely different challenge to Lillestrom and the media scrutiny had probably ratcheted up two or three notches at Stavanger, where there are three daily newspapers, each with at least two pages to fill on Viking. Then there was the national TV and national media, so we had six or seven journalists, plus TV crews and cameramen at every single training session. I had to speak with them every day, which helped me to learn how the media works and what you can and cannot say. It was all very much an open house and open-minded attitude, which is the Norwegian mentality and normal way of life.

We had raised the expectations to levels they hadn't been at for a number of years and now we'd have to try and kick on again. Viking hadn't won the league for 16 years so the supporters had become used to seeing their team not challenging for the title, but I think we rekindled some of that passion and hope – although that could also work against us if we didn't progress. By finishing third we'd also qualified for the UEFA Cup, so there was plenty to look forward to. We were playing in front of crowds of 16,000 at the Viking Stadion – about 7,000 more than we'd had in my final season at Lillestrom – so we had the backing from the people of Stavanger which was fantastic, and if we could channel the energy, enthusiasm and euphoria building up around the club, we'd be unstoppable.

The Royal League had been suspended due to financial problems, which was a pity – I thought it was a fantastic idea but when teams began putting weakened sides out, it was the death knell for the competition, which also had to battle against the Scandinavian winters. The sponsors pulled the plug because of falling attendances and viewing figures weren't anything like they'd hoped for. It was disappointing because I'd had a good experience in the competition with Lillestrom, and it gave you a ready-made competitive close-season programme.

So we had the Norwegian winter break as normal and we wouldn't compete in the UEFA Cup until the following July because our season ended so early in comparison with most of mainland Europe. Gunnar and I had hoped to build on that successful first season but our pre-season turned into a catas- trophe as one thing after another went wrong. Some of players, buoyed by unexpected success and media attention, thought they'd done enough to earn moves elsewhere and then our top scorer, Peter Ijeh, broke his pelvis, which was the biggest blow of all. We couldn't find a replacement for him because he'd been so prolific for us and, as everyone in football knows, goal- scorers are hard to find.

We missed Ijeh's goals badly. Had we had him fit all season, I think we could have challenged for the title. We tried to resolve the issue by spending some big money, but it would also prove a costly lesson for me. Unlike Lillestrom, the board at Viking felt that we were heading in the right direction and they proved it by giving me the finances to improve the squad. In search of a goalscorer, I signed Andrius Velicka, a Lithuanian striker from Hearts, for £1m. He'd scored 23 goals in 45 starts for Hearts and joined us in February in time for the 2008 campaign. He had a good track record, was powerfully built and seemed to be the answer to our problems up front – but he would prove to be anything but. After just four games, he told me he wanted to leave Viking because he and his wife couldn't settle in Norway and he couldn't continue. There was no more to be said of the situation – he wanted out.

I was aware that Glasgow Rangers had wanted to sign him but knew that Hearts would never have willingly sold him to a Scottish Premier League rival, so it was my theory – and nothing more – that Velicka used Viking as a stepping stone to get to the club he really wanted to play for. He made only a handful of appearances for us before the board accepted a £1m bid from Rangers. I felt we'd been used and let down by Velicka and I just couldn't believe the reasons he gave for wanting to leave Viking. His departure left us in a very difficult situation where we had to play, at times, without a recognised striker and it affected us markedly.

In Europe we squeezed past FK Vetra 2-1 over two legs but despite drawing 0-0 at Honka Espoo in the second qualifying round, we lost 2-1 at home to crash out of the UEFA Cup, which was a big disappointment for me and the club.

In summary, the season had started well and we topped the table after four games, but we were unpredictable and won just two of our next 10 games and dropped to tenth; then we lost just one of our next nine games to move back up to fifth. Our form was a bit up and down throughout the campaign. Though we hadn't reached the highs of the previous season, with maybe 10 minutes of the season remaining, a win would have given us a fourth-place finish in the table. As it was, we ended up losing 3-2 to Stromgodset to finish in sixth, on the same points as Rosenborg with the same goal difference but having scored fewer goals over the course of the season. I still believe we performed as well as we could without a recognised goalscorer for the majority of the season.

Our challenge for the title had not been anywhere near as strong as we'd hoped and Stabaek had run away with the championship, finishing 15 points above us. I could sense the media were turning against me and questions started to be asked about whether I was the right man to take the club forward. I couldn't risk another season of disappointment so, with an ageing squad, I decided it was time to shake things up a little, move some players on and bring in some fresh blood. We needed to build a new team because I felt I'd taken them as far as I could, so we began to rebuild. Some players were released, others offered new deals and we began bringing in some new faces.

On a personal level, 2008 was a horrendous year. My dad had slipped into a coma that he was in for 55 days before he died, aged 70, of massive organ failure. My mother had taken him away to celebrate his birthday and he collapsed of internal bleeding not long after he returned home. Then Hans Koziol, my trusted friend and agent, died that year and my grandfather, Hans, also passed away.

As if I'd not suffered enough, we then learned that my son, Tony, needed a serious operation to remove a tumour on his spleen. Thank God it was a cyst and not malignant, but he was only 11 and it was one of the most terrifying periods of my life. He came through with no complications, but it had been a terrible year and without doubt, it affected my work, too, because I was flying to and from Germany for several weeks

Pre-season didn't go too well and the unrest that had bubbled beneath the surface in the local press began to rise as the weeks progressed. Questions about some of the players we'd let go were asked, and I knew I was facing a battle to keep the local media on my side. Due to the inactivity over the winter, the pre-season games became the main focus and they were taken even more seriously than they had been a Lillestrom. There was live coverage of some matches and the games were treated as importantly as league fixtures. Whereas I believed pre-season was all about trying out new tactics, seeing how certain players performed and building up fitness, every game was treated as though more depended on them than it actually did. Damning conclusions and opinions were formed before our season had even started, and the newspapers even made tables based on our pre-season results, predicting what might lie ahead.

There was little I could do as the local journalists gradually turned on me and began giving me a hard time, knowing that unless we did something special, they wouldn't let up until they had got what they wanted. I had to try and get them back on my side. While I would always stand my ground and defend my players, the pressure grew as the season progressed and a succession of injuries and a general bedding of the younger players meant we weren't firing on all cylinders, which was to be expected as we went through a period of transition.

A parting of the ways became inevitable as we finished the season in 10th, just two points off sixth spot. I had signed a three-year contract extension before the start of the campaign, but I knew what was coming. The owner and the sporting director publicly backed me and were aware that I was trying to build a new team and that it would take time. Unfortunately, the supporters and press weren't prepared to wait any longer. The grass is always greener on the other side.

We were still getting crowds of 16,000 for our home matches, but the euphoric atmosphere had become a little negative and the atmosphere in town wasn't always very pleasant. As I said, Stavanger can be an intense place to live and doubly so when things aren't going your way. I recall one front page headline along the lines of 'Time for Rosler to go' and it was spotted by my son, Tony, who shouted: "Hey, Papa! Look, your picture is in the paper."

It was a tough time for my family because I was there to work and we had no support network. We noticed that when things didn't go well, people we thought of as friends became a little distant. By the end of the season, I met with the owner and sporting director, thanked them for all their public support and backing, which meant a lot to me, but that I thought it was in the best interests of all parties if I moved on. I duly had my contract cancelled by mutual consent, and my time in Stavanger was over.

I'd learned a lot with Viking and I'm glad I had the experience to manage them – even though I knew before I arrived that it had proved something of a managerial graveyard. I now needed to assess the past five years and take a step back and reflect. I'd jumped straight into management and wanted to become better at my job, so the best option was to take a little time out of the game.

# 23

# Kurze Begegnung

## (Brief encounter)

Now that I had a little more time on my hands, I accepted an invitation from Official City Supporters' Club, who were celebrating their 60th anniversary, requesting that I be their guest of honour. Once again, the club had been very generous and they paid for my hotel and flights. I went to the stadium with Cecilie where there was a big marquee set up underneath one of the stands.

We discovered we were sat on the top table with Chief Executive Officer Garry Cook, which was a pleasant surprise. Everyone was enjoying a big dinner and I was having a terrific evening. It was great to see a lot of my old team-mates. I think it was John Stapleton who was presenting the evening, and I was taken aback when a club official sat on our table informed me that I was going to be inducted into the Hall of Fame. I asked if he was serious and asked when this was supposed to happen, to which he calmly replied: "In five minutes." That's when I started to panic! I told Cecilie that I had to get a speech together quickly as I'd got nothing prepared. The next five minutes were a complete blur as I pretty much shut everything else out as I tried to get a few words down so as other people went up to the stage and spoke, I heard nothing.

Garry Cook was presenting my award and after a few words, I heard him say something along the lines of: "So it's my great pleasure to introduce Uwe Rosler into the Manchester United Hall of Fame..." As I was still focusing on my own speech, I didn't really understand what he'd said, but all of a sudden there was a lot of jeering towards Garry and I snapped out of my trance. I was a bit perturbed and asked Cecilie if they were booing me – but she explained what Garry had just said. I'd wondered if some of the City fans did not want me in the Hall of Fame after all.

I got up and said a few words, but there were still some City fans shouting at Garry, who must have wanted the ground to open up and swallow him. It was just a lapse in concentration and it could have happened to anyone, but of course, to City fans, it was as bad as it got! I didn't hold it against Garry and it's unfortunate that a lot of people won't forget that moment because he had been instrumental in bringing a lot of former players back to the club by looking after them, welcoming them and celebrating their part in MCFC history. I also think he was instrumental in the success the club has enjoyed recently and I hope that isn't forgotten. It was still a great honour for me and something I'm immensely proud of.

I returned home but didn't want to jump straight back into management, so I decided to take stock of my career and have a break. It was nothing more than a hiatus, but I felt after five years non-stop, now was the time to smoothen some of the rough edges I still felt I had. It was a gamble, because if you're out of the loop for too long, people wonder why and you can be quickly forgotten. It was a time to reflect, absorb new ideas and update my skills, so I began to travel around looking for new inspiration, as well as having some quality time with my wife and sons. We had a nice holiday and break around Christmas with the knowledge that I would begin my quest to learn more and become a better manager in the New Year.

So I headed to England, where I'd enjoyed my happiest time as a player, and started to watch games, training sessions and talk to various managers and coaches. I also travelled through-out Scandinavia and Germany because my long-term goal had always been to end up as a manager in England or Germany, though Denmark was also a possibility. I felt I'd done all I could in Norway because in Viking and Lillestrom, I'd managed two of the biggest clubs in the country – only Rosenborg were big-ger and I had no intention of managing them at the time.

Norway had been good to me and I'd thoroughly enjoyed my time there, both in the good times and bad. I'd met some great people and had the chance to learn my trade, so I couldn't have had a better grounding. I also knew that each club I'd been at had improved and were left stronger than when I'd arrived – both Lillestrom and Viking went into decline after Gunnar and I left, proving the theories of individuals and the press incor-rect, but I took no pleasure in that. I did think that, career-wise, another spell in Norwegian football would mean I wouldn't find any work outside the country in years to come as I'd be some-what pigeon-holed, so I had to make the break.

I also had the children to think of, too. They were at an age when they could still be moved relatively easily with minimal effect on their life. In another few years they'd have friends and social lives all of their own, so there was only a small window of opportunity to move on.

It was around this time that I started working for TV2 as a pundit for Norway's most popular football show. It was the Norwegian version of Sky Sports and I was invited on board by anchor-man Vegard Jansen Hagen as a specialist for the Premier League. I was told I could sell myself in a different way because I wasn't like other managers and maybe had an unusual outlook. They said I could learn about the media and the way it functioned from another angle, which might prove invaluable in the future, so I accepted the offer and began working for them, and I loved it. I really got into the analysis and tactical side of matches in the build-ups, at half-time and in post-match discussions of live games.

It was very educational, interesting and it allowed me to project myself in a way I hadn't been able to previously, especially in Norway, where I still think I was sometimes thought of as this crazy German guy. I'll always be indebted to Vegard for taking a chance on me and it was a role I would do for the next 18 months as I continued to travel around. It would also give me a much-needed income during my time out of football.

In England I would network, make contacts and get my name in the frame for one or two things because I knew jobs wouldn't just land at my feet. I would stay in England for maybe 10 days of every month and I couldn't have done it without the help of two close friends, Peter Beagrie and Gary Lee. I lived at Gary's place and sometimes with Beags and his family, hired a car and travelled around. I was able to come and go as I pleased. I went to Blackpool, Sunderland, Bury and Port Vale to watch games and training. Beags opened a lot of doors for me as I travelled around. I also watched City train, went to the Academy and spoke with coaches. I then went to my place in Majorca and watched Real Mallorca train every day for two weeks. Then I travelled to Germany and went to Hoffenheim – where Ralph Rangnick was head coach – and studied their training and methods. All of this helped me look at the way I'd been managing in a different light. It gave me ideas and sessions that I took note of for future use. I also did a management leadership course in Stavanger in a bid to improve myself and I felt I was learning all the time.

Then, fate played a hand as we came to England as a family for a short break over Easter in 2010. We came to watch City play and I recall that we couldn't fly back to Norway because an ash cloud from an Icelandic volcano eruption had grounded planes all over Europe. We had to stay an extra 10 days before we could get a flight home and it was during this time that we decided that, actually, we didn't want to leave. We'd had a good time and we felt at home and it felt like the right thing for me and my family to do, so we made plans to move back to England permanently. I knew the level and standard required in English football, and also accepted I wouldn't get a job in the Premier League or Championship – but League One or League Two, at the very least, were a possibility.

However, it would prove a frustrating time as I applied for a number of jobs but didn't even make the shortlist for an interview at any of them. Clearly, it was going to be even harder than I'd imagined, but at least I was welcomed back by City with open arms. Garry Cook had helped us with the move from Norway and had made it clear that I was very welcome at the club where, under the new ownership, they wanted to re-establish the club's traditions and welcome old players back into the fore. I was invited on trips to represent the club in an ambassadorial role and I always felt very welcome and proud to be associated with City once again. Garry, who I can only speak in glowing terms about, arranged for the club's welfare officer, Des Coffey, an old friend of mine who had organised my English lessons during my early days at City, to sort out an interview at Cheadle Hulme School to get my kids in. We wanted to live in Bramhall, which was an area we'd always loved, and though my kids spoke English, they couldn't write it, and the school had very high standards. Although Tony was fine, we had to get a tutor for Colin but within a couple of months, he had caught up, as kids do.

The school term began in September and by then, the plan was to be settled in England in a new home. We'd sold our home in Lillestrom and our apartment in Stavanger and we rented a home in Wilmslow for six months while we hunted for our new home. But there was to be one final twist and it turned out Norwegian football was to offer me one last challenge.

On 16 August, 2010, the day we packed our belongings to leave Stavanger, I received a call asking if I would be interested in taking on a job at Molde. I didn't hesitate in accepting, though I wanted the position purely on a temporary basis. Molde had finished as runners-up in the league the season before and now they were third-from-bottom and looking as though they may be relegated. So I called Gunnar and told him we had to take the job. I met with the sporting director and he told me what Molde needed and I was pleased they had thought of me. I probably wasn't the most popular figure in Norwegian football because of my reputation for being outspoken and had said one or two things that had ruffled a few feathers.

I hadn't been very wise with some of things I'd said and had probably upset one or two of the main journalists along the way – which is never a good idea! Molde knew that they had to stay up because 2011 was their 125th anniversary, and celebrating from the second tier of Norwegian football would have been a dampener to say the least. The remit was simple – keep the club up. I think it's fair to say that Molde had lined up Ole Gunnar Solskjaer for the 2011 season, but I assume he wouldn't have come if the club had been relegated, so there was a lot at stake.

I made a deal. My family moved to England as planned, while I stayed and managed Molde for three months and then I left, regardless of the outcome. Gunnar and I had eight games to save Molde, who hadn't won for 10 games and were third-from-bottom – so no pressure, then!

There was an international break underway when I took over. The sporting director told me that a team-building exercise had been planned a few days after I arrived, and did I want to continue with it? I was happy to do so. It was the perfect opportunity for me to gauge the mood of the squad and the characters I'd be depending on in the coming weeks. So we headed for a fjord to stay at an army barracks for three nights, where we would also play a friendly match.

We split the squad into three groups, each had a coach as its leader and we had to do everything with them. We did shooting, scrambling through a storm drain, climbing, running and crossing rivers and we had to do everything as a team, helping each other and depending on one another. Then, in the evening, we had a barbecue and a few beers and they must have thought, 'Maybe this guy is okay' – but the whole point was to let everyone relax while allowing me to get to know them well in a different environment. After that, the ice was broken, the team spirit was fantastic and we went from strength to strength.

My first game was against Stromgodset who we beat 3-1 away from home, and then followed that up with a 1-0 win over Honefoss. We secured a 1-1 draw at Lillestrom, a 2-0 home win over Kongsvinger and a 1-0 victory at Tromso. We ended with a 0-0 draw at home to Odd Grenland, a 1-0 win at Haugesund and completed the season with a 1-0 home success over Stabaek. Six wins and two draws from eight games – it was better than the form of champions, Rosenborg, and I knew we'd turned that club around with some simple fine-tuning, a few players brought back into the team and a few left out, plus a more productive formation and a change in the mind-set of the players.

We improved the discipline and professionalism of the squad and we did a good job. Once I'd convinced the players that perhaps the persona of me painted in the media wasn't how I actually was in reality, everything worked like clockwork. I was still battling against things I'd done five years ago when I'd been at Lillestrom, and I suppose people don't forget characters who, on occasion, think or act outside of the box.

I had a wonderful time at Molde and at the end of the season I had to give a speech in front of our home fans. They gave Gunnar and I a standing ovation and I knew they'd really taken us to their hearts. The sporting director even came to me and asked me if I wanted to stay on. I told him that I'd loved it, but we had an agreement and that's what I wanted to stick by. Everything had turned out exactly as I had hoped it would and it brought my time in Norway to a very positive conclusion.

The players, supporters and even the media had taken to me, but I think my decision to leave made things easy for him if truth be told because I'm convinced Ole Gunnar Solskjaer was already lined up – he was a hero in Norway, so I suppose if I was paving the way for anyone, I was glad it was him.

Now it was time to follow my family and see what the future had in store for us in England. I asked Gunnar if he would be interested in joining me in England, if and when I found work, and he just said: "Let's see" – and we agreed to just leave it there and see what happened.

It was the first time I'd ever lived apart from my family and now I was looking forward to being reunited with them to start our new life in England.

# 24

# London ruft

## (London calling)

It felt good to be back in England and now there was just one thing missing – a job. I had to get my name into the frame when positions became available but I had no track record here, and I doubt people knew of my time in Norway. Of course, it would all be down on my CV, but unless I actually had the chance to speak to somebody, I couldn't express my enthusiasm or explain my management style.

Peter Beagrie was a massive help at this stage. He was commentating for Sky Sports and he took me with him when he went to matches and would take me into the managers' offices so I could network, meet new people and put myself in the mind of clubs if and when vacancies came up. Beags opened a lot of doors for me and he took me to places like Barnsley, Sunderland and Hull City – where my old gaffer, Brian Horton, was – and a host of other clubs.

I was taking in as many matches as I could as we went into December 2010. I watched Port Vale a number of times and Bradford City, too, where Beags was a former player and coach and knew the people who made decisions. Both clubs were close to where we were living and they were in League One and League Two, which were the two divisions I'd targeted. Bradford's manager, Peter Taylor, was under a lot of pressure and if they replaced him at any point, I wanted to know as much about the players and the style of football they played so that if I applied, the board would know I'd done my homework.

In between, I caught other games all over the north of England and when a vacancy came up at Port Vale, I put my CV in and hoped for the best. Jim Gannon had been sacked and I thought I knew enough about Vale to at least get an interview. I also applied for a vacancy at Walsall and then the Bradford job became available. Bury was another option, but my application for the post at Bradford and Port Vale must have barely registered, with only Walsall having the decency to send me a letter thanking me for my interest.

In the meantime, I spent time at City's Academy where my son, Colin, had been taken into the shadow squad before being moved up to the squad for his age level. I was a regular attendee at Platt Lane – so much so that the head of coaching, Scott Sellars, asked me if I was interested in doing anything on the coaching side. He knew my background in Norway and asked if I fancied working with the strikers from the ages of 16 to 19. We made an agreement that I would take three 45-minute sessions per week with the strikers and I could choose the content of the sessions. It was great because I was keeping myself involved as well as learning how City's Academy operated. I watched Scott and Steve Eyre take sessions and I learned a lot because they are both excellent coaches. I started watching a lot of Under-18 and Under-21 games in addition to the lower league matches I was still taking in. It was a great experience and around April, Scott asked me, hypothetically, if a job became available, would I be interested in taking on the role of City's Under-18s coach? It was tempting, but my burning desire was to manage a Football League club – that's where I felt I was most effective.

I really enjoy working with young players and developing them, but I've always been in an environment that needed to produce results first and foremost, which is totally different from how academies work where, quite rightly, development matters more than results.

City intend to be the best academy in the world and to work there, you have to be a specialist in the coaching of young kids. That is the reason I said I wouldn't apply if a position came up. Would I have got the job if I'd have applied? I'm not sure, but I appreciated Scott thinking of me.

The 2010/11 season ended and I was still no nearer to finding a job than when I had first arrived in November. Then, finally, my agent managed to set up an interview at Bury and I thought this may at last be my chance. I was to go and meet the board at 5pm, so I went to the Four Seasons Hotel in Hale with my agent and Peter Farrell, the former first-team coach at Bolton Wanderers, and someone I'd got to know during my travels around the north. Peter and I had met a few times at different games and then hooked up and had proper discussions on football which I found very interesting. He started going to games and doing match reports for me and I went to games and gave him feedback. As we were both looking to get back into the game, we helped each other out and as he was also a coaching assessor for the FA, I thought he was someone who could be part of my coaching team, if and when I found gainful employment. We got along well and he was very knowledgeable about all levels of English football.

We'd prepared down to the last detail for the interview and then a few hours before we were due to leave, Bury cancelled the interview. I was devastated, and that was the lowest I'd felt in six months of job hunting. I hadn't even come close to getting the job at Bury, despite my experience as a manager in Norway, which was a relatively much higher level than League Two. I started to wonder if I would ever find work in England and felt completely lost. In Norway, I'd usually been approached to be the manager and then it was down to me to sell myself to the club, but I wasn't even getting the chance to do that here, where 70-80 applicants chased each job. Seemingly if you had no experience in England, then forget it.

I wasn't sure where to go from here, so I couldn't believe what happened next. I received a phone call from my agent asking me if I would like to have an interview with Brentford in League One, where Andy Scott had been sacked. I instantly agreed, but then he added that the interview was in two days' time.

"Two days? I've never seen them play."

Of course, there was no question of me not making that interview so I had to organise myself – and quickly. Paul Dickov was manager at Oldham Athletic at the time and his team had recently played Brentford, so he helped me out by supplying three DVDs. My agent then got me another, so I had four to study ahead of the meeting.

I prepared myself as well as I could and spoke to people in the game who had seen them play, such as Peter Beagrie, and then tried to put a good case together to be their new manager. I met with Andrew Mills, the CEO at the time, and things had seemed to go well. He was very knowledgeable about football, but I went away not knowing if I had impressed him or not. I was surprised that he left the club soon after that, but he must have recommended me because I then received a call to arrange a meeting with owner Matthew Benham and his right-hand man, and we seemed to get on well with each other. He was looking for someone who thought outside the box, and he didn't want a typical English manager as such.

The first question he asked me was whether I was familiar with the model of having a sporting director and could I work with one if I was? Of course, I'd worked with a sporting director at Lillestrom, Viking and Molde, and it was all I'd known, so I said I absolutely didn't have a problem with that, so long as the roles were absolutely clear and our jobs defined to the letter and written down. I told Matthew I was more or less driven to work with a sporting director and that I saw my role as managing the first-team and everything connected with it. I said I'd need an Academy director who would work along the guidelines we'd put in place for the senior side. I would then allow them to get on with their job because I had no intention of overseeing the Academy.

I think Matthew liked that when he heard it and so he interviewed me further a few days later, which again seemed to go well. Then I was interviewed by Frank McParland, who is the

Academy director at Liverpool and a close friend of the owner. He asked me very specific football questions such as the structure I would put in place, what was my philosophy, whether I liked working with younger or older players, what type of pay structure I would implement, whether I wanted results immediately or preferred to develop a team and he also gave me a number of hypothetical situations to discover how I would deal with them. He was very honest and open with me and I needed to be precise and concrete with my answers because he was a clever man. If I'd been trying to wing anything, he would have picked up on it straight away.

Matthew had wanted to test me with a few different interviews and situations in order to get the best for Brentford Football Club and I had no problem with that. My fourth interview was with the owner again, during which we began to negotiate a potential contract. I still hadn't been given the green light that I'd actually got the job, and I was very keen to get all possible scenarios with the sporting director down in writing because past experience had taught me that things could go positively or not so good.

It took two weeks to hammer out all the small print – who signed the players, who did this, who did that – most of which I did over the phone from Germany. Even during that period I think Derek McInnes was interviewed and I also heard Martin Allen's name mentioned for the job – but as far as I knew, I was still in the box-seat.

I was travelling down to London on the train and received a phone call from a journalist saying he'd heard I was the new manager. I didn't know what he'd been told, or by whom, so I had to deny things and hold back because I didn't know for sure. Finally, the owner asked me to meet with the sporting director, Mark Warburton, to see if we had any chemistry. So we met at Wembley and by that time, I knew Mark had applied for the manager's job because he'd been assistant-manager when Nicky Forster had taken on the Brentford job on a caretaker basis until the end of the season. Mark was quite close to the owner and had also been Academy director of Watford, so he was clearly a smart guy.

We had never met each other before and I felt a little awkward knowing that he had wanted to be manager. However, I had put the feelers out about him from the contacts I had in the game and the feedback I had about him was very good. I was a little reserved at the meeting and held back a little because I didn't want to give too much away. I think Mark was the same, so it wasn't the easiest of meetings, and of all the interviews I'd had up to that point, that was the first one where I left feeling that things hadn't gone very well.

I'm not sure what Mark fed back to the owner, but in spite of my concerns, it must have been good because I was finally offered the job which, of course, I was delighted to accept. Agreeing terms wasn't a problem because it was never about money – just about having the opportunity to prove myself in English football as a manager. I fully accepted that and was happy that the owner trusted me and had faith in me to manage his club.

The first call I made was to Gunnar Halle in Norway, but he told me the timing wasn't good as his kids were at a special age in their schooling and he couldn't uproot them. I completely understood his reasons and though it would be a little strange not to have him alongside me, I was delighted that Peter Farrell accepted the offer of becoming my first-team coach. The new season was on the horizon – just two weeks away in fact – so Mark and I began working straight away on the squad.

I then found out something interesting not long after I'd started. Our owner was the founder of the NextGen Under-21 tournament in which big European clubs competed in group stages. For the tournament, he'd wanted a Norwegian club to take part, so he called Ole Gunnar Solskjaer at Molde, soon after he'd taken the job on, to see if he would be willing to enter a side. Matthew sent representatives over to convince Ole Gunnar to agree and during a discussion between the pair, Ole Gunnar asked Matthew if he was looking for a new manager?

He said he was, and Ole Gunnar said: "Why not try Uwe Rosler. He did a very good job at Molde and is very experienced in Norway. I highly recommend him."

That, I believe, was the key for me. I had already applied for the Brentford job along with 70 or 80 others. I know I would never have even got an interview had Ole Gunnar not spoken so highly of me. That's sometimes how life works and I owe Ole Gunnar a big thank you for what he said because he hadn't needed to do that – indeed, we don't even know each other that well. But all I had to do now was deliver on my promises...

# 25

# Bettwäsche in

## (Bedding in)

I was determined not to uproot my family again so I made the decision to commute to London from our home in Bramhall, staying most of the week in London with the odd day here and there at home. It wouldn't be easy because apart from those few months when I'd managed Molde, we'd never been apart. But I didn't want to take Tony and Colin out of school and as a family, we were settled.

I had so much energy and couldn't wait for the season to begin. With the owner's blessing, our sporting director Mark Warburton brought in several members of support staff from Watford who he knew well and trusted. Watford had lost their Premier League status and were having to make some massive cut-backs and we were the beneficiaries, inheriting some guys at the top of their profession, all of which was great news for Brentford and for me. The head of medical, head of analysis and head of conditioning all joined us from Watford and together their expertise and professionalism lifted our club to a new level. They were all Mark's department, and because the new season was almost upon us, I had a lot of meetings to get to know the new guys and make sure we were all working towards the same goals. We were all new to the club; they didn't know how I worked and vice versa, so there was a lot of organising still to do.

I discovered in a very short time that all the new guys were top quality and a real asset to our football club. I decided very quickly to give the relevant responsibility to the head of medical because these guys didn't need anyone to tell them what to do. It's my belief we have one of the best medical departments outside the Premier League and probably better than a good number of top-level sides, too.

It was a challenging but exciting working environment and we styled the fitness department to match the style of football we wanted to play. I showed our fitness coach exactly what I wanted, and he got it immediately. He then took it to another level, so again, I had these dedicated, talented guys working around me, and as a manager, I really couldn't have asked for any more. I was able to concentrate on the players and get to know their strengths and what sort of characters they had, as well as dealing with agents, which was a whole new ball game for me.

In Norway there were just three or four agents and everyone tried to get on with each other but, in England, there are so many – and here it's all about the money. Of course, there are some good agents out there, but you also have individuals who are not interested in the welfare of the club or their clients – just their cut in the deal. With those sorts, it's not about a career-plan for their player, just what their percentage will be.

My working relationship with Mark Warburton developed rapidly to a very trusting, forward thinking and energetic operation. His knowledge of younger players around the country enabled us to forge strong links with clubs like Everton and Southampton, and it helped us change the structure of our team. We changed the squad completely and from the 16 players I inherited from the previous manager, after one year there was nobody left from the previous regime, other than those we'd re-signed, younger players we'd promoted to the senior squad and new arrivals.

I inherited a very honest, hard-working group of players with a lot of experience. They were mostly in their mid-to-late twenties and if I'd have carried on with them, we'd have always been safe in that we'd never be relegated, but never quite good enough to push for promotion. We'd continue as 'safe' Brentford – a club who knew their place in League One, doing what was expected of them and no more. I felt we had to aspire for more and so did the owner and Mark Warburton.

Matthew Benham wanted to see his club promoted, and he asked me if I could achieve it on the budget he'd given me. I said that it would be difficult, but that we'd give it a go. We were competing against teams like Sheffield Wednesday, Sheffield United, Preston North End, Charlton Athletic and Huddersfield Town – not to mention Bournemouth, who had a new, wealthy owner, plus others – all clubs with better squads on paper and bigger transfer budgets.

I think the Brentford fans were a little sceptical in the beginning in regards to my appointment. I think it's fair to say they initially may have preferred someone like Martin Allen, who had taken them to the play-offs, and perhaps gone with someone more tried and trusted – and English. They knew about Uwe Rosler as a player, but as a manager, I was an unknown quantity to them and, in many ways, something of a gamble. Norwegian football means little to English fans so there was a certain amount of pessimism that I had to overcome. I needed to prove myself to them, which was perfectly understandable.

The owner said he wasn't too worried about promotion in the first season – he just wanted to see better football. He had been very disillusioned – in his words – with the football that had been played for the previous few seasons so my first challenge was to change the style of football and to do that, I had to change the players. I needed talented players who would be good on the ball and very fit, plus a professional attitude after coming from a professional environment.

Not every League One player came from professional environments so our philosophy to achieve our aims was to go for younger players from bigger clubs on loan. We had excellent support staff that could look after the players to Premier League levels and, meanwhile, they would be playing a style of football that would help them develop and gain vital experience, too. Those were our basic aims and it worked out fantastically well for us.

I had always felt our coaching team was one man short and intended to bring in an assistant-manager, in addition to first-team coach, Peter Farrell. Alan Kernaghan, a former teammate at City, had always remained a friend to me and we had kept in touch over the years. He ticked a lot of the boxes regarding the sort of person I was looking for to enhance our team. Two months before the end of my first season, I asked him to join us for the last few matches as a sort of trial to see if we could possibly work well together, and I was delighted that he accepted the offer. His contribution was very important in those final weeks with his professionalism, energy, enthusiasm and knowledge giving us a real lift which helped us achieve our goals for that season.

I think our supporters started to warm to me from our very first game onwards because the style of football was different and better to watch. Even though I'd inherited a squad rather than built one from scratch, everyone bought into the new ideas set by myself and Mark, and the fitness and medical departments. There was a positive atmosphere, the football improved and the supporters could see what we were trying to achieve. We weren't perfect and it didn't always work, but our intent was to play the game the right way and it made for a very enjoyable first year in charge at Griffin Park. However, there was one incident that left a bad taste in my mouth, something that maybe cost us a play-off place and who knows, maybe promotion, too.

Not long before the run-in towards the end of the season, we were in a very promising position to make a late surge into the play-off places. We'd been in the top 10 consistently for most of the season and I felt we could find the momentum we needed in the remaining games to finish in the top six. So it was extremely disappointing when our on-going contract negotiations with our top scorer, Gary Alexander, broke down. His current deal expired in the summer and we'd offered him a one-year extension, with very realistic targets to reach to secure a second year in terms of the number of games he would need to play. He was reliable and I enjoyed working with him because Gary was a leader in the dressing room and a very positive person who could be relied upon when he went out on the pitch. He'd really enjoyed the season and had found a rich vein of goalscoring form, which was a bonus because while he had always been a hard-working player throughout his career, he'd never been a prolific scorer and his goals might just have been the difference on the run-in.

We'd managed him throughout the season because he had an on-going knee problem, and with treatment and training to suit his rehab, he was available for almost every game. I was enjoying working with him and everything was going as well as I could have hoped. Then, around March time, I received a phone call from Mark Warburton, warning me that Gary was going to call me. I was watching my son Colin train at City's Academy and I took the call from Gary not long after.

He told me that he wanted to leave the club. I almost laughed it off because the timing was so odd, having come completely out of the blue.

"You can't go now, we still have a chance of making the play-offs," I told him.

"I want to leave and I want to now," he said, and I could sense he was becoming agitated.

"Gary, you have a contract and I can't let you go."

What came next effectively ended any relationship I had with him and he made his position untenable at Brentford. He put me in a position where I could never allow him to play for me or the club again and, frankly, I was disgusted with his attitude. I'd never come across anything like this before in almost six years of management and I hope it never happens again.

Between Gary and his agent, they seemingly bullied their way to a move and there was no way back for him, which is probably what he'd intended from the beginning. He'd crossed the line with what he said to me and went way beyond what any player should say to his manager. I couldn't have felt any more let down than I did.

I told Mark to let him go and he signed for Crawley Town, initially on loan, with the promise of a two-year contract to follow. It was a lot closer to his home, which was on the other side of London, and financially a more secure contract for him and his family, but it left us without our leading scorer at the worst possible time. It was very difficult to replace Gary because there was just a week before the loan window closed and, ultimately, I think the cost to Brentford was huge. I know he did what he did for his family and I think that he is a decent bloke, but what he did and said was unforgiveable.

I couldn't tell our supporters exactly what had happened, and instead gave a watered down account of what had occurred and wished Gary all the best. I know people were mystified why we'd allowed him to go, but I had to take it on the chin until the dust settled. I think our fans read between the lines because they're not daft, but they didn't know the whole story.

I believe that as a direct result, we lost our next three games because the lads felt they had lost someone who was going to be pivotal to our hopes. We couldn't have timed our worst run of the season at a more inopportune time.

We pressed on and brought in Clinton Morrison on loan from Sheffield Wednesday. He helped give everyone a lift because everyone was deflated when the news broke about Gary, with people muttering that we had no chance now he'd gone. Clint wasn't 100 per cent match fit, which is why we'd been able to get him, but I'd been happy to take the gamble. We rediscovered our form, winning five games in a row then drawing a couple, but with three games to go, we played Stevenage, who were our main rivals for sixth position. If we won, we'd go above them by one point into sixth. It was our cup final and with the score at 0-0, we won a penalty which Sam Saunders missed. Then we were awarded another spot-kick and Clayton Donaldson missed his effort – it was as if someone up above didn't want us to win that game. Inevitably, Stevenage went ahead, then increased their lead to 2-0 as we went searching for an equaliser. We pulled one back straight away – but we couldn't find a second and lost 2-1. The result meant our challenge was effectively over. Our regular penalty taker that season had, of course, been Gary Alexander.

I had always felt that if we had our key players fit, we'd have had a great chance, but I can't help but think that we'd definitely have made the play-offs with Gary in our team. We were the side that looked as though we would just sneak in just as another side ran out of steam – it happens every year, so it proved a frustrating finish.

After the season had ended, I got a call from Gary, but I didn't answer it. I know he's still in regular contact with some of my staff, which is absolutely fine and I do understand his motives – it was just the way he went about things that disappointed me.

We finished our first season just three points shy of the play-off positions, the club's best finish for seven years. I'd learned a lot about the league and managing in England and the whole season had been a massive learning curve for me, which would only hold me in good stead for my second season and for Brentford. Bringing in Alan Kernaghan had worked really well, and he accepted a permanent position on our coaching staff, which I now felt was complete. The question was, could we improve again and maybe go one better for the 2012/13 season?

# 26

# Fußball kann ein grausames Spiel sein...

## (Football can be a cruel game...)

Both myself and Mark Warburton wanted to raise the bar for our second season. We'd achieved the target we'd been set in the first year by finishing in the top 10, but we wanted to kick on again. Our minimum target for the new season, set by the board and the owner, was to finish in the play-off positions and take it from there. We knew it would be tough, but what a year it would prove to be, memorable for so many reasons – even if we did have something of a rollercoaster finish to the campaign.

We wanted to bring in some new talent and when I looked back to Gary Alexander's departure, I actually thought it might have turned out to be a good thing for all concerned. If we'd have given him the two-year deal he wanted so badly, it might have actually held us back because we were looking to move in a different direction.

We started the campaign off by going to Germany for pre-season training, while the calibre of players we were bringing in was also adding more quality to the squad. I was able to spend money for the first time and we brought in Tony Craig, a left-back from Millwall, who I always felt could also play as a left centre-half. I watched him a number of times and had seen him fill in at central-half a number of times, so I felt he could do a job for us in that role.

People were starting to sit up and take notice of Brentford because we'd been shown on Sky a number of times the previous season. We always played good football and we were getting a reputation for being an attractive League One side. We'd played Huddersfield Town live on TV and completely outplayed them – but we lost 3-2 after leading 2-0, I felt partly due to a couple of controversial refereeing decisions that cost us dearly. We'd also played Charlton Athletic and won 3-0 at The Valley, so our reputation was growing. Suddenly people were trying to make things difficult for us in the transfer market where we were being tagged as 'big spending Brentford', which was a total inaccuracy.

The perception was that we were wealthy and it became harder and harder to complete some deals due to the image that we, for some reason, had acquired. The assumption was that we were a London club and we'd improved so much because we'd brought a lot of new players in so we must have wealth – but that assertion was untrue because we'd had exactly the same budget for two years running. Some former managers didn't help by spreading rumours in the media about what we were paying our players, in comparison to other clubs in our division.

One thing we had done though, was to change our pay structure by trimming the squad from 24 professionals to 19 established players. By doing that, we saved some money and were able to pay our top performers a little bit more, while keeping well within our budget.

This approach also made it a little easier to bring players to Brentford. We trimmed the squad by releasing or moving on players who would never play for me, and we introduced a pyramid wage system. There were players who were in the highest band and two further tiers, which reflected where each individual was at that time. It was all down to good housekeeping and nothing more, plus good use of the loan system which saw us form a fantastic relationship with several Premier League sides, and Everton in particular.

Mark Warburton had excellent contacts with the Everton Academy and I developed a really good relationship with David Moyes. It saw Adam Forshaw and Jake Bidwell come to Brentford, and we had players arrive from Fulham, Southampton and Norwich City, too. It meant we could bring in top quality youngsters for relatively little outlay – and that was our secret. Our philosophy was to offer upcoming young players their first loan spell in League football.

Because we were a League One side, we wouldn't be able to afford to bring in players who were having their second or third loan deal because they would have already shown their quality by then and become too expensive for us. We'd bring them in on a three, six or 12-month loan deal, and then offer to make the deal permanent, if possible. The infrastructure and ambition of the club means that we can develop players and offer them first-team football, while and in return give the parent club a huge sell-on fee – that's the price of getting in that kind of quality. However, it's a small price to pay in reality, and Brentford are the main beneficiaries in the long term. While we think we have a very good system for bringing in young players, by contrast, we have found it really hard to bring in more experienced players on the budget we have – but that is something we will deal with.

Whereas the first season saw us enter the play-off positions on a few occasions, we spent virtually the whole of the 2012/13 season in the top six – and a lot of time in the top two, with our consistency and quality excellent all season. We would also have a really good FA Cup run, which turned into a big money-making machine. Our two high-profile games against Chelsea brought in a lot of revenue and gave our players the opportunity to show what they were capable of over two games against the European champions. If that didn't give us confidence to kick on, I didn't know what would.

One thing I can always promise is that my teams will always be physically strong at the end of the season. Our mentality may have been something we needed to look at, but from a fitness point of view, we'd always be there until the end. While some teams would begin to wilt, we would become stronger. All season long I would ask the players, 'can we make the last game of the season a final and win promotion on our own ground?' That was always our mind-set and even if we had a hiccup along the way, we'd say okay, it's not a problem – we can still achieve our goal.

I was quite sure we could make the play-offs, but I believed we could also win automatic promotion. Throughout the whole season it was as though we were following a script – everything was perfect. Even the problems we had with agents, injuries and suspensions couldn't knock us out of our stride, and just as we'd planned all season, we went into the final game of the season at Griffin Park knowing a win over Doncaster Rovers would mean we would be promoted. It was perfect.

The build-up to the match was incredible, with media hype surrounding the match unbelievable. Fortunately, we were well prepared because the two games against Chelsea had been equally manic. If questions were asked of our club, we came through each challenge with flying colours, from the big press conferences to handling the media accreditation and the requests of not just the local journalists, but for those from The Sun, The Daily Mirror and The Times. It felt like the football world was focused on Brentford FC and our players and I think everyone handled the situation superbly.

As the manager, I had to decide the preparation and it wasn't easy. Did we go to a hotel or just treat it as a normal match? I believed it was our time and that we were absolutely ready for this. We had the best home record in the division, playing against a team whose momentum was on a slightly downward curve and we felt we held all the aces.

We knew it wasn't going to be easy because Doncaster were defensively very strong, and they arrived knowing a draw would win them promotion. And that's exactly how they set out – with the intention of seeing through the job and leaving with a 0-0 result because they had no interest in trying to win the game. They sat deep, and it was hard for us to break through a packed midfield and defence where Doncaster were strong and tall. We struggled to break them down and continually had them under pressure. Sometimes you get the break, and sometimes you don't – and we did in the form of a 94th-minute penalty. The scenario had been perfect – and now it was too perfect. The whole season had gone exactly to plan and now, with virtually the last kick of the game, we had a penalty that could send us up into the Championship.

As soon as the referee pointed to the spot, our whole bench jumped up and the supporters went crazy, starting to celebrate as though we'd won promotion. In an instant, I knew we wouldn't score. I screamed to my coach and players: "What the fuck are you doing? Are you crazy?" I was absolutely furious because we had nothing to celebrate and, of course, we then missed the penalty, the ball coming back out off the crossbar.

The referee was waiting for the ball to go into touch so he could blow for full-time. It got cleared to the halfway line where one of their players just happened to be standing. They then went up the other end and within something like 10 seconds, the ball was in our net and we'd lost 1-0. I think the gods had been watching us and, had we stayed calm and waited until after the penalty was taken, I think that, somehow, things would have gone our way. Of course, then there is the story behind the penalty-kick and for that I will need to backtrack a little.

Our budget had been spent but because we'd made money against Chelsea, we were able to bring Bradley Wright-Phillips in for the last two months of the season, which gave us a lift. Under normal circumstances we couldn't have afforded him. Unfortunately, we had several problems in the remaining weeks that were no fault of our own. Liam Moore, a centre-half, had been brought in on a three-month loan from Leicester City but despite a verbal agreement with his parent club, that he would stay with us and play first-team football until the last kick of the season, we had lost him two days before the transfer window closed. Liam was very successful for us and played all the games, but Leicester recalled him which went totally against the agreement we'd made. Their captain had picked up a suspension, which meant they needed defensive cover, but we suffered as a result.

We had six games to go and just two fit centre-halves to see us through. I was devastated by the way Leicester behaved because we'd kept our part of the bargain – but they didn't keep theirs. They were entitled to do what they did, but it wasn't how I would conduct my business. I also felt sorry for Liam, who loved playing for us and didn't want to go back. It was a mess.

Then our goalkeeper situation reached crisis point, too, with our first-choice goalkeeper, Simon Moore, struggling with an ongoing hip problem. He couldn't train because he had to rest after each game, and our second choice, Richard Lee, had aggravated a shoulder injury we originally thought we'd had under control. Our only other option was Antoine Gounet, a French goalkeeper who was a little short of experience in League football and it would have been unfair to pitch him in at such a critical stage of the season. We'd used up all our aces as we entered the final strait and we would have to patch up the walking wounded and hope that we limped over the line with the squad we had.

We went to promotion-rivals Sheffield United with just two centre-halves, and Tony Craig was shown a red card for violent conduct, which we would unsuccessfully appeal against – so we had to put club captain Kevin O'Connor in there as cover. O'Connor was a dependable and long-serving Brentford player who had picked up a long-term injury early on in my first season, and then had another lengthy spell on the sidelines in my second year. He'd hardly played for five months but was a very reliable player and a fantastic person. In that game, Marcello Trotta, on loan from Fulham, converted a penalty for us, so he probably thought he was the man for the job if the situation arose again in the remaining weeks.

O'Connor had been our regular penalty-taker – at least he had been in the years before I arrived – but because he'd hardly played, he'd never taken one for me. We'd missed a lot of penalties during the season and, as noted, the previous season we'd missed spot-kicks at Stevenage that had potentially cost us a place in the play-offs, so I wanted someone experienced to take one if we were awarded a penalty against Doncaster. I asked Kevin what he thought, and he told me he'd only missed two out of 20 or so penalties in his career, so I said, 'Okay, I want you to take it.' I told the team that he would take the penalty if we were awarded one but perhaps I didn't make it 110 per cent clear to everyone. I should have maybe written it on the wall, and told Sam Saunders and Marcello Trotta again before the game, but I didn't.

Kevin practiced taking penalties in the days leading up to the Doncaster game and, of course, with the score at 0-0, we were awarded a penalty deep into injury-time. Kevin slowly started to walk towards the area and, in the meantime, I saw two or three of our lads by the penalty spot in discussion, presumably about who was going to take it. Clayton Donaldson, Sam Saunders and Marcello Trotta were all around the ball and I felt something was wrong. I then shouted to the lads to make sure Kevin took it.

Of course, we'd found ourselves in a unique, almost once in a lifetime situation, with so much at stake and promotion just one kick away. Marcello, full of belief in his own ability and having scored against Sheffield United, was confident he could do it again, and Kevin, as ever wanting the best for Brentford, could see this was neither the time nor the place to create a fuss. He then asked Marcello if he was sure, and was told: "Yes, of course." So he allowed Marcello to continue. His shot hit the bar and the dream had ended by no more than a coat of paint.

Looking back, I admire Marcello for having the guts to do what he thought was the right thing to do at that moment, and for Kevin to have the guts to do what he felt was the right thing to do for the team and the football club. Nobody is to blame for the penalty not being converted – it was just a moment we didn't get right collectively, though everyone had Brentford's best interests at heart.

# 27

# Zurück von den Toten

## (Back from the dead)

The whole club was devastated and I've never felt lower in football. In the dressing room there were a lot of tears, some because they knew that they would never get that close to playing in the Championship again, and there were the younger lads who had worked their nuts off all season and were mentally spent. It was awful.

People wrote us off saying that we were gone, mentally, and that we wouldn't be able to pick ourselves up in time for the play-off semi-final – but they didn't understand the heart, spirit and determination my group of players have.

The day after, we had the end-of-season dinner and my first thought was to cancel it. But then I changed my mind, believing it was absolutely the right thing to do. Marcello had taken so much stick that he didn't want to come, but eventually we persuaded him to attend and I'm glad he did. We were still in the play-offs and so we had to start picking ourselves up.

When he arrived, me and Mark Warburton spoke to him for 15 minutes and we cleared one or two things up, and things went really well. The whole team looked after Marcello and our fans were fantastic. I knew there and then that we were going to be alright. We had a good night, a few beers and everyone loosened up. The mood quickly changed from anger and frustration to determination. The ending hadn't been written yet, and though it had felt like our world had caved in, we had to start focusing on the fact we still had a route to promotion.

We were to play Swindon Town over two legs on the Saturday and the following Monday, and had a week to prepare. We had got ourselves back on our feet despite everyone expecting us to be mentally spent, and we went to the County Ground for the first leg in good heart. Typically, after what had happened against Doncaster, we were awarded a penalty and this time there was no doubt about the taker – Kevin O'Connor, filling in again at centre-half, smacked the ball home and we drew 1-1 with it all still to do at Griffin Park.

Jonathan Douglas, one of our best players over the previous two seasons, had played with a knee injury for the last two months of the season and only surgery would fix the issue. He would play, but then he had to rest because he couldn't train as well. He played in the first leg but with another game coming up so quickly, I knew there would have to be changes in a number of positions if we were to go into the second game as fresh as possible.

Players like Douglas were typical of the never-say-die attitude we had among our lads, who were willing to do anything for Brentford. Now we had yet another massive home game, with the media focus firmly on our club. It was Chelsea and Doncaster all over again, and we'd pack out Griffin Park to capacity for the second leg – I think we hadn't sold out a game before the season for something like 25 years, and now we'd done it three times in the space of two months! Everyone wondered if we could hold our nerve after what had happened, especially with Wembley and the possibility of promotion as the prize.

As for team selection for the second leg, I had some massive calls to make – and one of them was recalling Marcello Trotta. Considering what had happened the last time we had played at home, it as a huge gamble, but I had confidence in him and admired his courage, so I had no doubt he'd be okay. We had a strong squad and everyone was fit – apart from Douglas, who had a niggling knee injury – while Swindon had a smaller squad than us, and had to play with the same team they had started with 48 hours earlier.

The advantage we had was that I could bring in four or five new faces to energise our side and one of them was Trotta, but at the same time I also had to rest Jonathan Douglas because he hadn't had enough time to recover. It was the first time we'd played without him in such a huge game and it was a gamble, but as the game wore on, we were looking fantastic and were 3-1 up with 75 minutes gone – so what happened next was crazy because in the whole season, we hadn't conceded one goal from a corner in the first phase, so this was a bad time to do exactly that in this game. Incredibly, Swindon scored again in the last minute to force extra-time – it was torture and yet again we were having to do things the hard way.

In extra-time Swindon had a man sent off and we had plenty of chances to win the game, but we just couldn't find the winner, which meant penalties again – it was unbelievable. We'd missed two against Stevenage to miss out on the play-offs in my first season, we'd missed one against Doncaster on the final day to miss out on promotion – surely fate couldn't be that cruel a third time? Imagine the mental strength my players needed going into a penalty shoot-out with all the baggage we, as a club, were carrying with us.

We still had a job to do so I got the lads together and asked who wanted to take a penalty. Some did and some didn't, but I still felt it was our destiny to win so I was fairly relaxed about everything. I was sure we would win, even though we'd lost a 3-1 lead during 90 minutes. I hadn't been sure against Doncaster, but I did now because I believed it was our fate.

The younger lads took responsibility on the day and things couldn't have gone better as Swindon missed one of their spot-kicks but we scored all five – the relief was incredible in the stadium, and we now faced yet another huge game with a final at Wembley against Yeovil Town. What we'd achieved that season, I felt, was to give our fans yet another showpiece game. We'd had two against Chelsea, the Doncaster match and two epic ties with Swindon Town. It was unprecedented for our supporters, but we had to see the job through.

Yet again, the question was how to approach such a massive occasion. I was angry that there was now a gap of 13 days until the final, after being forced to play back-to-back semis in such a short space of time. All the hard work the players had put in over the 10 long months would boil down to just one 90-minute game with so much at stake – and it made no sense. My concern was, how could we possibly keep our rhythm going until we faced Yeovil? The momentum we would have taken into the final had it been played a few days later would, I believe, have carried us over the line, but now we had to figure out how to plan what happened in-between. Did we give the players some time off, take them away, organise a training camp, play a friendly?

It was very difficult for me to plan and even more so because I had some terrible news at home, where Cecilie lost the baby we were expecting. That overshadowed everything else because I needed to be there for my wife, just as she'd been there for me every step of the way when I needed her – yet we also had this massive game to contend with. Typically, Cecilie was as strong as ever and insisted I saw this period through, but although we decided to take the lads away to Cardiff for a three-day training camp, I stayed at home with my wife.

I returned five days before the final and we played an internal game at Griffin Park. It was then that I decided not to play Jonathan Douglas – one of the hardest management decisions I've ever had to do. I felt the team had done so well against Swindon in such a high-pressure game that I wanted to start with the same players in the final. Jonathan had given everything for me whenever he'd been called upon, and was a fantastic and integral part of the club – but I couldn't risk him at Wembley as he was still carrying a knock. I already had Simon Moore and Harry Forrester, who were borderline with their fitness, so we were already pushing it. The truth was, if anyone deserved to play, it was Jonathan, but I had to pick a team that I believed would give us the best chance of winning.

Jonathan was devastated and I completely understood why,

but I had to do what I thought was right for the club. I had to let the lads get on with it while I stayed at home with Cecilie, but I returned just before the final. We stayed at a hotel prior to the final and tried to keep things as low key as normal, but of course, heading into a game at Wembley, things are anything but normal. For some of the lads, it's a once in a lifetime game but I felt we had an edge over Yeovil because we had played in the Johnstone's Paint Trophy a few months before I arrived, plus I felt that we had enough experience of big games to handle this one. Our one problem was that they were a bit of a bogey team for us.

The game itself began badly and they opened the scoring with a world-class strike from Paddy Madden after just six minutes. Simon Moore could do nothing about it, and all credit to him for scoring what was the goal of a lifetime. But for us, it was the worst possible start. After that, we settled into the match and started to put pressure on them but crucially, we didn't score and they were looking dangerous on the break.

Then, almost on half-time, they scored again. We had conceded from a second phase corner again – our third in three games – proving that we clearly didn't have enough height at the back. We had to change things around because we were 2-0 down and the game was slipping away from us.

The plan had always been to bring Jonathan on in the second half. I thought we'd be leading by that stage and he would be able to shore things up at the back and help take us over the line. The situation meant I couldn't bring him on because we were now chasing the game, so we made one or two tactical changes and completely dominated the second half, pulling a goal back almost straight away through Harlee Dean, and then had two or three massive chances, a couple which fell to Bradley Wright-Phillips, but we just couldn't find the equaliser and lost the game 2-1.

Looking back, there are many things that can go against you in a big game like that. Sometimes you just don't turn up, you can freeze on the day or you don't get the rub of the green – anything can happen on the day. Their goalkeeper was Man of the Match, which speaks volumes for how much possession we had and how many chances we created. Unfortunately, the bottom line was that our moment was against Doncaster and it just didn't happen for us. I was very disappointed but I felt emotionally drained, with the games we'd had and losing the baby.

I was glad the season was over and that I could spend some quality time with my family. Cecilie and I just disappeared to America for a few days on our own. Looking back, people will say it was a disappointing season but I think it was a great 10 months, and it is unfair to suggest it was anything other than that.

What I found really encouraging was that at the end of the game at Wembley, the owner came into the dressing room and asked me if he could say a few words. It wasn't planned, and I was more than happy for him to speak. He told everyone that he really wanted to have a go during the 2013/14 season, having gone so close, and that is what we all needed to hear because we'd just had another slug in the guts, even though it had been a fantastic campaign with so many highs.

Brentford were approached by a Championship club and a foreign club during the summer but I had no intentions of leaving the club at that time and though we made a tricky start to the new season, we soon put together a run that once again saw us challenging for promotion in what was a harder League One than ever before.

As far as I was concerned, everything was on track and the lads had picked themselves up after the play-off final hangover against Yeovil and things couldn't have been going better.

But living in Bramhall and working in London was difficult on a number of levels so when Wigan Athletic offered me the chance to manage in the Championship – plus the opportunity to be at home with my wife and sons every night, it was too good an opportunity to turn down.

I knew I was leaving Brentford in excellent shape and I was delighted Mark Warburton was given the chance to take the club on and he's picked up the reins and continued the fine work we all did together and, all being well, the club will achieve promotion ahead of schedule. I'll forever be indebted to Brentford, the owner and the supporters for giving me the chance to manage in England and I leave behind only happy memories and good wishes.

Wigan Athletic offered me the chance to test myself at a higher level. The club is geared for Premier League football and the goal is to take the club back to where it belongs as quickly as possible. We have an excellent squad of players, a passionate chairman and a great set of supporters. Everyone has responded superbly since I arrived.

I hope there are many more chapters to be written for both myself and Wigan Athletic.

# Index

# INDEX

# UWE ROSLER

# INDEX

# INDEX

# INDEX

# Statistics

## Playing Career – Club

| Club | Period |
|---|---|
| 1. FC Lokomotive Leipzig | 1982-1988 |
| BSG Chemie Leipzig (loan) | 1988-1989 |
| 1. FC Magdeburg | 1989-1990 |
| Dynamo Dresden | 1990-1992 |
| 1. FC Nurnberg | 1992-1994 |
| Dynamo Dresden (loan) | 1993-1994 |
| Manchester City | 1994-1998 |
| Kaiserslautern | 1998-1999 |
| Berliner Tennis Club Borussia | 1999-2000 |
| Southampton | 2000-2002 |
| West Bromwich Albion (loan) | 2001 |
| Spielvereinigung Unterhaching | 2002 |
| Lillestrom | 2002-2003 |

## Seaon-by-season record

### East Germany

| Season | Club | Division | App | Gls |
|---|---|---|---|---|
| 1987–88 | Lokomotive Leipzig | DDR-Oberliga | 6 | 0 |
| 1988–89 | Chemie Leipzig | DDR-Liga | 27 | 6 |
| 1988–89 | Magdeburg | DDR-Oberliga | 9 | 3 |
| 1989–90 | Magdeburg | DDR-Oberliga | 24 | 11 |
| 1990–91 | Magdeburg | NOFV-Oberliga | 17 | 5 |
| 1990–91 | Dynamo Dresden | NOFV-Oberliga | 15 | 3 |

# UWE ROSLER

## Germany

| Season | Club | Division | App | Gls |
|---|---|---|---|---|
| 1991–92 | Dynamo Dresden | Bundesliga | 36 | 6 |
| 1992–93 | Nürnberg | Bundesliga | 31 | 3 |
| 1993–94 | Dynamo Dresden | Bundesliga | 8 | 0 |

## England

| | | | | |
|---|---|---|---|---|
| 1993–94 | Manchester City | Premiership | 12 | 5 |
| 1994–95 | Manchester City | Premiership | 38 | 22 |
| 1995–96 | Manchester City | Premiership | 44 | 13 |
| 1996–97 | Manchester City | Division One | 49 | 17 |
| 1997–98 | Manchester City | Division One | 33 | 7 |

## Germany

| | | | | |
|---|---|---|---|---|
| 1998–99 | Kaiserslautern | Bundesliga | 37 | 12 |
| 1999–2000 | Tennis Borussia Berlin | 2. Bundesliga | 30 | 9 |

## England

| | | | | |
|---|---|---|---|---|
| 2000–01 | Southampton | Premiership | 24 | 1 |
| 2001–02 | Southampton | Premiership | 5 | 0 |
| 2001–02 | West Bromwich Albion | Division One | 5 | 1 |

## Germany

| | | | | |
|---|---|---|---|---|
| 2001–02 | SpVgg Unterhaching | 2. Bundesliga | 14 | 5 |

## Norway

| | | | | |
|---|---|---|---|---|
| 2002 | Lillestrøm | Tippeligaen | 12 | 9 |
| 2003 | Lillestrøm | Tippeligaen | 1 | 1 |

## Totals

| Country | App | Gls |
|---|---|---|
| East Germany | 98 | 28 |
| Germany | 156 | 35 |
| England | 210 | 66 |
| Norway | 13 | 10 |
| **Career total** | **477** | **139** |

# STATISTICS

## **Playing Career – International**

East Germany                    1990        5 caps

| Date | Opposition | Venue | Result |
|------|-----------|-------|--------|
| Jan 26, 1990 | Kuwait | Kuwait | W2-1 |
| Mar 3, 1990 | United States | Berlin | W3-2 |
| Apr 11, 1990 | Egypt | Karl-Mark-Stadt | W2-0 |
| May 13, 1990 | Brazil | Rio de Janeiro | D3-3 |
| Sep 12, 1990 | Belgium | Brussels | W2-0 |

| Played | Won | Drawn | Lost | For | Against |
|--------|-----|-------|------|-----|---------|
| 5 | 4 | 1 | 0 | 12 | 6 |

## **Managerial Career**

| Club | Period |
|------|--------|
| Lillestrom | Nov 1, 2004 – Nov 13, 2006 |
| Viking Stavanger | Nov 22, 2006 – Nov 18, 2009 |
| Molde | Aug 30, 2010 – Dec 31, 2010 |
| Brentford | June 10, 2011 – Dec 7, 2013 |
| Wigan Athletic | Dec 7, 2013 – present |

## **Record in Norway**

| | Games | Won | Drawn | Lost | Win % |
|---|-------|-----|-------|------|-------|
| Lillestrom | 55 | 24 | 16 | 15 | 43.64% |
| Viking | 89 | 37 | 24 | 28 | 41.57% |
| Molde | 8 | 6 | 2 | 0 | 75.00% |

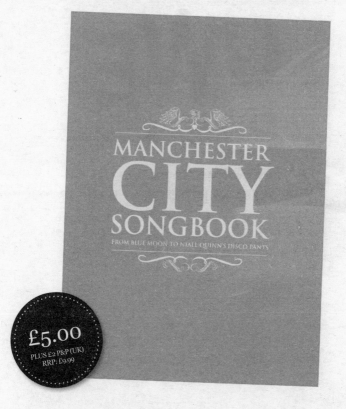 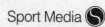

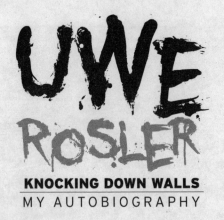

# UWE ROSLER

## KNOCKING DOWN WALLS

### MY AUTOBIOGRAPHY